Post-Stroke Rehabilitation

Edited by Pratap Sanchetee

Published in London, United Kingdom

Post-Stroke Rehabilitation
http://dx.doi.org/10.5772/intechopen.98083
Edited by Pratap Sanchetee

Contributors
Mohammad Shaikhul Hasan, Kanida Narattharaksha, Nahar Afrin, Md. Sazzad Hossain, Iria Beltrán Rodríguez, Óscar Durán-Borrella, Patricia González-Feito, Rebeca de la Fuente Blanco, Irene Sánchez Serrano, Laura García-Talavera Casado, Mubarak Muhammad, Rabi'U Musa Isah, Abdurrazak Muhammad, Fahad Somaa, Sabarisah Hashim, Mahaneem Mohamed, Mustapha Muzaimi, Che Mohd Nasril Che Mohd Nassir, Khaidatul Akmar Kamaruzaman, Mohd Haniff Abu Zarim, Sanihah Abdul Halim, Paulina Ortega Bastidas, Pablo Aqueveque, Britam Arom Gomez, Karen Barriga, Francisco Saavedra, Polycarp Nwoha, Florence Osita Okoro, Emmanuel Nwoha, Augustine Obi, Chidinma Oluchi Nwoha, Iyanu Ayoola, Nkeiru Christiana Ogoko, Peace Ngozi Nwoha, Catherine Wali, Anna Idaguko, Nnenna Chinagozi-Amanze, Ifeoma H. Nwoha-Okpara, Pratap Sanchetee

First published in London, United Kingdom, 2022 by IntechOpen
IntechOpen is the global imprint of INTECHOPEN LIMITED, registered in England and Wales, registration number: 11086078, 5 Princes Gate Court, London, SW7 2QJ, United Kingdom

British Library Cataloguing-in-Publication Data
A catalogue record for this book is available from the British Library

Additional hard and PDF copies can be obtained from orders@intechopen.com

Post-Stroke Rehabilitation
Edited by Pratap Sanchetee
p. cm.
Print ISBN 978-1-80355-351-1
Online ISBN 978-1-80355-352-8
eBook (PDF) ISBN 978-1-80355-353-5

Meet the editor

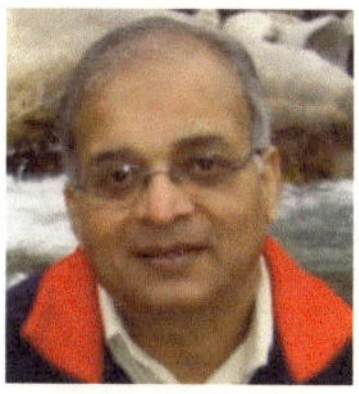

Dr. Pratap Sanchetee obtained MBBS from *Dr. Sampurnanand Medical College*, India in 1970. He obtained an MD from the University of Rajasthan, India in 1974, and a DM in Neurology from the Postgraduate Institute of Medical Education & Research (PGIMER), Chandigarh, India in 1985. He served in the Armed Forces India as a physician and neurologist for twenty-four years and retired as a Lieutenant Colonel in 1998. During 1994–1998, he also served as an Associate Professor at the Armed Forces Medical College, Pune, India. He received the Chief of the Army Staff Commendation in 1980. Since 1998, he has been pursuing clinical practice in neurology at various hospitals in Jodhpur and Guwahati Assam. He is a visiting professor, Ph.D. guide, and advisor to Jain Visva Bharti University (JVBI) and Bhagwan Mahaveer International Research Centre (BMIRC), Ladnun, Rajasthan. He is the Director of Research at the Spiritual Training Research Foundation (STRF), Mumbai, India. His areas of interest include the mind as an interface between the soul and body, meditation and brain, and delivery of neurology care in society. Dr. Sanchetee is a lifetime member of nine national associations. He is the editor of four books and has published 110 original papers, chapters, and review articles in national and international journals. He was associated with the "Tropical Neurology Subsection" of the Indian Academy of Neurology as Chairperson and Secretary for more than ten years. He regularly participates in national and international conferences. Dr. Sanchetee was executive editor of the *Medical Journal Armed Forces India and Journal of Indian Academy of Geriatrics.*

Contents

Preface

Stroke is a major public health issue and its prevalence is increasing as the aging population increases. Despite the best treatment available, 30%–50% of stroke survivors are left with significant physical and/or psychological disabilities and consequent decline in quality of life. Neurorehabilitation is an established standard of care for improving functional capabilities and quality of life following a stroke. A good rehabilitation schedule can result in substantial recovery in up to 80% of cases. Stroke rehabilitation is a multidisciplinary approach involving physicians or stroke specialists, nurses, physiotherapists, psychologists, nutritionists, occupational therapists, speech therapists, and audiologists. However, there is a shortage of neurorehabilitation programs across the globe, more so in resource-poor countries. This book covers widespread topics related to stroke rehabilitation during both the acute and chronic phases. Experts in the field discuss not only medical aspects but also issues of patients and community participation. The book also addresses cognitive deficits and psychological problems faced by patients and their caregivers.

The field of stroke rehabilitation has a bright future. Despite the good potential for recovery, rehabilitative measures are underutilized. Major barriers to their implementation include limited availability, geographical distance, high cost, and lack of awareness about their benefits. This book is a comprehensive reference that includes the latest knowledge and practical guidance on the subject. There is a requirement to develop low-cost tools that will have high acceptance among patients and caregivers. To maintain the continuum for stroke care and reduce morbidity and mortality, there is a need for public health systems in both developed and developing countries to improve stroke awareness and to implement proper strategies of triage, acute treatment, well-defined rehabilitation plans, and teleservices.

This book is a useful resource for all those connected with stroke care including physicians, physiotherapists, and rehabilitative specialists.

Dr. Pratap Sanchetee, MD, DM (Neurology)
Consultant Neurologist,
Sanchetee Neurology Research Institute,
Jodhpur, Rajasthan, India

Section 1

Rehabilitation

Chapter 1

Post-Stroke Rehabilitation: A Necessary Step

Iria Beltrán-Rodríguez, Laura García-Talavera Casado, Óscar Durán-Borrella, Patricia González-Feito, Irene Sánchez-Serrano and Rebeca de la Fuente Blanco

Abstract

A stroke is defined by the abrupt and sudden onset of neurological signs and symptoms that occur due to a disorder in cerebral blood circulation. Cerebrovascular diseases are a well-known cause of morbidity and mortality, being the second cause of mortality and disability throughout the world. Stroke treatment has improved substantially in recent years with the implementation of stroke units and revascularization therapies. The role of rehabilitation is to help improve deficits to regain functionality and to define the needs and care in patients with permanent disabilities. Stroke rehabilitation must start early and intensively and it must be carried out by a multidisciplinary team made up of neurologists, rehabilitation doctors, nurses, physiotherapists, occupational therapists, speech therapists, neuropsychologists, neurophysiologists, and social workers. Patients and families should be actively involved with this team, if possible, from the beginning and throughout the rehabilitation process. Functional recovery through comprehensive rehabilitation allows patients to remain in their usual environment, perform their work duties and carry out activities of daily life by themselves, reducing the need for institutionalization in long-term care facilities.

Keywords: stroke, rehabilitation, disability, skills, recovery

1. Introduction

A stroke is defined by the abrupt and sudden onset of neurological signs and symptoms that occur due to a disorder in cerebral blood circulation. It can be due to an excess of blood in the cranial cavity, which is in expansible, called hemorrhagic stroke; or due to insufficient blood supply of oxygen and nutrients to the parenchyma: an ischemic stroke. Strokes usually have symptoms related to a focal brain lesion, an abrupt onset followed by stabilization with a tendency to regress, and predisposing risk factors.

We should suspect it when the following symptoms suddenly appear: weakness or numbness of a half body; difficulty speaking or understanding language; vision difficulty in one or both eyes having ruled out ophthalmological pathology, vertigo, or instability associated with other neurological symptoms or signs.

Cerebrovascular diseases are the second cause of morbidity and mortality in the world [1].

There is an estimated prevalence of about 80 million people with stroke worldwide. In 2016, of the 80.1 million affected, 41.1 were women and 39 were men [1].

The highest risk of stroke is found in populations in East Asia, Central Europe, and Eastern Europe. In terms of race, the incidence per 100.000 inhabitants of ischemic stroke is higher in black than in Hispanic, and higher in Hispanic than in white; being all the etiologies of stroke more frequent in black, except cardioembolic [2, 3].

In the last 30 years, a decrease in the incidence and mortality from stroke has been observed due to the better control of vascular risk factors, health education, and advances in the treatment of the acute phase of stroke. This improvement, unfortunately, is not universal and is highly influenced by the economic situation and the educational background of the population in each geographic area. In recent years, a decrease in the incidence of stroke has been observed in whites, remaining constant in blacks [4].

Hand in hand with the global decrease in incidence and mortality rates is the increase in the prevalence of stroke and its social health impact, due to a longer life expectancy and increased survival rate of patients suffering from cerebrovascular events.

Stroke patients have a high risk of poor prognosis during the first year after the event, including rehospitalization (33%), recurrence (7–13%), dementia (7–23%), mild cognitive disorder (35–47%), depression (30–50%) and fatigue (35–92%), all contributing to affect health-related quality of life [5, 6].

Stroke units and revascularization therapies have changed the stroke prognosis [7]. The role of rehabilitation is to help improve deficits, regain functionality and define the needs and care in patients with permanent disabilities. Disability in stroke varies according to the initial severity, the location of the injury, the patient's pre-morbid state, the degree of neurological recovery, and the support system that surrounds the patient [7, 8].

It is evidenced that comprehensive rehabilitation after stroke has a prognostic impact that is maintained in the long term, in the form of a better functional situation for the patients who access it. Functional recovery through comprehensive rehabilitation allows patients to remain in their usual environment, perform their work duties and carry out activities of daily life autonomously, reducing the need for institutionalization in long-term care facilities [9].

The recommendations of the King's College research team, in collaboration with the European Alliance Against Stroke, which presented the document "*The impact of stroke in Europe to the European Parliament*", indicate that multidisciplinary evaluations should be carried out in the stroke unit and the rehabilitation should start as soon as the patient is medically stable. People who start rehabilitation within the first week after admission have better long-term results than those who start their rehabilitation later [10].

2. Stroke rhabilitation

2.1 Pathophysiology and principles of neurological rehabilitation

The cells of the nervous system and the endothelial cells are continuously interacting with each other and with the extracellular matrix in order to maintain continuous cerebral homeostasis, forming a functional unit called the neurovascular unit. It is made up of neurons, interneurons, astrocytes, basal lamina lined with smooth muscle cells and pericytes, endothelial cells, and an extracellular matrix [11]. All these elements, interconnected with each other, constitute a highly efficient system for regulating cerebral blood flow [11]. Cerebrovascular events alter the correct molecular communication between each of the elements of the neurovascular unit, generating a functional dysregulation that leads to the damage of the tissue. In the functional recovery phase after an ischemic stroke, compensatory neurovascular signaling at this level favors the repair mechanisms that involve angiogenesis and neurogenesis, thus intervening in achieving the most complete functional recovery possible [12].

Astrocytes play a fundamental role in cerebrovascular events, both in the establishment of the definitive lesion and in the process of tissue repair. During ischemia, the first morphological change observed is the edema of astrocytes, being one of the responsible factors for the decrease in glutamate reuptake. The edema may be surrounding the lesion up to 8 weeks after the stroke, which may alter the functioning of nearby neurons by blocking neuronal conduction [10].

Glial cells that survive the ischemic episode undergo a process of hypertrophy and proliferation, known as reactive gliosis, which has been related to mechanisms of neuroprotection and repair of ischemic injuries [13].

Recovery after stroke is associated with cortical reorganization [8]. After a cerebrovascular event, the tissue recovery that takes place during weeks, months, or years after the acute event is related to different physiological phenomena: dendritic growth, formation of new synapses (synaptogenesis), functional reorganization in the injured area or participation of other neighboring or homologous areas of the contralateral hemisphere in the process. These phenomena can occur spontaneously and they can be facilitated and directed by rehabilitative therapeutic interventions [13].

In ischemic stroke, the obstruction of a cerebral artery generates local changes in cerebral blood flow (CBF). Under normal conditions, CBF through adult brain tissue is >50 ml/100 g of brain parenchyma/minute. When the CBF is reduced in a certain area of the brain below 10 ml/100 g/min, a severe cerebral dysfunction is produced. This leads to a complete neuronal, structural and functional loss in that location in a short time; it is called the core of the infarction. Between this nucleus of ischemic infarction and the normally perfused brain parenchyma, there is a moderately vascularized region, the extent of which depends on the functioning of the collateral circulation, called the penumbra zone, in which two zones with different prognosis are differentiated: oligohemia zone (22–0 ml/100 g/min) and ischemic penumbra zone (10–22 ml/100 g/min) [14, 15]. The oligohemia zone is a hypoperfused zone that still maintains its functionality, while the ischemic penumbra is a hypoperfused and functionally inactive zone that limits the edges of the infarcted area but is still viable if CBF is recovered early [11]. Current strategies for acute reperfusion in ischemic stroke are aimed at restoring cerebral perfusion in the ischemic penumbra [11]. The therapeutic window in ischemic stroke is the time that elapses between the onset of ischemia and the moment in which the neuron located in the ischemic penumbra loses its ability to survive. After this time, reperfusion of the ischemic zone will be useless [13].

The tissue that survives a cerebrovascular event has the ability to adapt and reorganize itself anatomically and functionally to rebuild or replace synaptic connections that have been injured and reinforce neural networks that have remained after injury. This phenomenon is known as neuroplasticity [15], and neurological rehabilitation therapies play a fundamental role in its enhancement [16]. The key to activating neuronal plasticity is the repetition of the affected function, so all those treatment techniques that favor the performance of a function and its repetition will promote brain plasticity and the recovery of patients [9, 10].

The functional reassignment of the different healthy cortical areas to supply the deficit in the damaged area is called brain remapping [12].

The neuroanatomical, neurochemical, and functional changes that occur during the reorganization by neuroplasticity will facilitate, in some cases, the recovery of the affected functions (adaptive neuroplasticity). On other occasions, as a consequence of this reorganization in favor of some functions, the development of others may be hindered (maladaptive neuroplasticity) [17].

The most important cortical functions are not linked to specific anatomical regions, but rather depend on neural networks made up of neurons of diverse cortical locations interconnected with each other and distributed throughout the cerebral cortex [15, 18].

Although some functions of a neural network are specifically ascribed to a region of the same (e.g.: the execution of language to Broca's area), the lesion in that specific area may have little clinical translation if the remaining structures that makeup that network take over functional relief and thus compensate for the defect.

If the damage to a functional system is partial, recovery within the system itself is possible. On the other hand, if the damage is complete, replacement by a functionally related system is the only alternative for the functional recovery of the injured area. Each of the mechanisms involved in the post-injury functional recovery process will depend on the magnitude of the brain damage [16].

Although the basic mechanisms of neuroplasticity are common to the entire cerebral cortex, the pattern of cortical reorganization in the functional recovery of the different capacities is not the same, and the peculiarities in these patterns support the different modalities of therapeutic intervention for the different deficits: motor, sensory and cognitive (**Table 1**) [17, 19].

Motor recovery is a complex process that combines intrinsic or spontaneous neurological recovery and functional recovery. Intrinsic neurological recovery is the recovery of normal movement patterns, being the severity of the initial deficit inversely proportional to the recovery prognosis. It occurs generally within the first 1–3 months after the event. Functional recovery is the regaining of basic tasks or activities of daily life through learned compensatory movements (new movement patterns), which depends on motivation, learning capacity, family support, and the quality and intensity of the rehabilitative therapy [8].

The structures that help restore motor activity and function after a brain injury can be gathered into three groups: intact perilesional areas of the ipsilateral

Mechanisms of plasticity in neural networks	Mechanisms of plasticity in synapse
Recovery of neuronal excitability	Changes in intracellular signaling
Activation of neural pathways partially unscathed	Generation of axonal sprouting and dendritic from uninjured collaterals
Plasticity with assembly type neurons	Axonal regeneration
Synaptic unmasking dependent on neural activity.	Unmasking of networks previously existing but functionally inactive
Recruitment of neural network components	Long-term potentiation
Modulation by neurotransmitters of the excitability of subnetworks.	Long-term depression

Table 1.
Mechanisms of neuroplasticity [19].

primary motor cortex, ipsilateral and contralesionally auxiliary motor systems together with the structures responsible for executive control and contralateral motor system [20].

In addition to neuroplasticity phenomena, the post-injury recovery process involves mechanisms of regeneration, differentiation, and maturation of new neurons and support cells that facilitate the creation of new neural networks, thus allowing the replacement of damaged ones [16]. Neurogenesis, gliogenesis, and angiogenesis refer to the development and formation of new neurons, supporting glial cells, and blood vessels respectively [14, 15]. Neurogenesis takes place throughout life, although it is attenuated with age. In adults, it is discrete and basically restricted to two neurogenic areas: the subventricular zone close to the third ventricle and the infragranular area of the dentate gyrus of the hippocampus [15]. Several studies have shown that ischemic lesions of the central nervous system lead to an increase in the proliferation of neural stem cells located in the subventricular zone, which will subsequently differentiate into mature cells that will travel to the damaged brain areas through different biochemical mechanisms and molecular cell signaling. Neuronal death is a strong stimulus for neurogenesis after ischemic stroke, even when it occurs in brain territories that are located at a distance from neurogenic niches. However, the vast majority of these newly generated cells have low survival once they reach the damaged area, a fact that could be favored by detrimental factors in the perilesional environment, lack of neurotrophic support, and molecular signaling which is necessary for proper development [16].

Both in the phenomena of neuroplasticity and cell regeneration, epigenetic regulation through mechanisms that include DNA methylation, histone modification and the action of micro-RNAs (miRNA) play a fundamental role [16].

2.2 Disability measurement scales

2.2.1 Disability of basic activities of daily living

2.2.1.1 Barthel scale

The most widely used and the fastest index of functional independence. Its completion time is 5 min. The maximum score is 100 points (complete functional independence for activities of daily living) and a score below 20 points will show a great dependency level. It rates the level of dependency with feeding, movement, personal grooming, getting on and off the toilet, bathing, walking on a level surface, ascend and descend stairs, dressing and undressing, and bowel and bladder continence [21].

2.2.1.2 Functional Independence Measure (FIM)

Assesses physical and cognitive disability according to the level of assistance required to carry out activities of daily life. Its completion time is 30–40 min. It consists of 18 items that assess 6 areas of function that are summarized in 2 basic domains: physical and cognitive. Each item scores on a scale of 1–7 (1 = total dependence and 7 = total independence), with a maximum score of 126 points. An unfavorable prognostic factor of function is considered a score less than 40 or a score less than 60 in people older than 75 years [9].

2.2.2 Motor disability

2.2.2.1 Motor index

It is a simple, fast scale: its completion time is 5 min and it is useful to assess voluntary motor activity in three basic movements of the upper limb (shoulder abduction, elbow flexion, and handgrip) and another three in the lower limb (hip flexion, knee extension, and foot dorsiflexion). 0 represents total paralysis and 100 represents normality [9].

2.2.2.2 Fugl-Meyer scale

It is used to assess the function and control of the musculoskeletal system, including balance, sensitivity, and joint pain in patients who have suffered a stroke. It has the disadvantage that it requires training for the evaluators, and its application is very slow, taking about 30–40 min. It consists of 155 items, each of which is scored on a three-point ordinal scale. The maximum motor performance score is 66 points for the upper limb, 34 points for the lower limb, 14 points for balance, 24 points for sensitivity, and 44 points each for passive joint movement and joint pain. A maximum of 266 points can be reached [9, 10].

2.2.3 Cognitive disability

2.2.3.1 Mini Mental State Examination (MMSE)

It is a brief test for the detection and quantitative evaluation of cognitive impairment. Its maximum score is 30 and the threshold value for cognitive impairment is 23. It consists of 11 questions that assess orientation in time and space, fixation, attention and calculation, memory, nomination, repetition, understanding, reading, writing, and replication of a drawing. The test is valid as a screening tool and is sensitive to detect moderate/severe impairment, but not mild impairment [10].

2.2.3.2 Montreal Cognitive Assessment (MoCA)

It is a short test that can be performed in 12 min to detect mild cognitive impairment. It consists of 30 questions, the score ranges from 0 to 30. A score above 26 is considered normal. It evaluates different types of cognitive abilities, including orientation, short-term memory, delayed recovery, executive function, visuospatial ability, language skills, abstraction, object naming, and attention [22].

2.2.4 Disability for communication

2.2.4.1 Boston aphasia test

It requires 1–4 h to do and consists of 16 slides for the diagnosis of aphasia and 60 graphic elements for the vocabulary test. 1 point is awarded for each correct answer, the maximum score being 60. A score above 50 is considered normal [23].

2.2.5 Walking disability

2.2.5.1 Sagunto Hospital Functional Gait Categories

Sagunto Hospital Functional Gait Categories (FACHS) allows a quick, valid, sensitive, and reliable assessment of ambulation, allowing to determine the walking speed of stroke patients. It has 6 self-exclusive and self-explanatory function levels. Level 0: impossible; 1: completely dependent; 2: dependent hand; 3: free; 4: prolonged and 5: normal [10].

2.2.6 Stroke severity

2.2.6.1 Modified Rankin scale

It is a scale to measure functional outcomes in post-stroke patients. Assigns a score of 1–5 based on the level of independence from pre-stroke activities. 0: Asymptomatic; 1: No significant disability, able to carry out all usual duties and activities; 2: Mild disability, unable to carry out all previous activities but able to look after own activities without assistance; 3: Moderate disability, requiring some help, but able to walk without assistance; 4: Moderately severe disability, unable to walk and to attend to own bodily needs without assistance; 5: Severe disability: bedridden, incontinent, and requiring constant nursing care and attention [24].

2.2.6.2 National Institutes of Health Stroke Scale (NIHSS)

It is a measure of somatosensory function used in the acute phase with patients who have suffered a stroke. It is made up of 11 items: level of consciousness, conjugate look, visual fields, facial paresis, paresis of upper extremities, lower extremity paresis, limb ataxia, sensitivity, language, dysarthria, extinction/neglect/inattention. It determines the severity of the stroke: Mild <4, Moderate <16, Severe <25, Very severe ≥25 [10].

2.2.6.3 Canadian Neurological Scale (CNS)

It is also used in the acute phase to assess the neurological status of stroke patients. Ten clinical domains are measured, including mental state: level of consciousness, orientation, language, and motor functions: face, proximal arm, distal arm, leg [10].

2.3 Upper and lower limb motor rehabilitation

Stroke is one of the main causes of disability in adults, and the demand for rehabilitation services after suffering a cerebrovascular event is very high.

Motor deficit is the main cause of physical disability in stroke and the area in which rehabilitation works as a priority. It is usually unilateral, although in more severe patients bilaterally innervated muscle functions, such as trunk control, may be affected [25, 26].

Hemiparesis or hemiplegia is the most prevalent deficit in stroke, being the symptom that is more worrying for the patient and their relatives, and the main indicator of treatment expectations [27]. The rehabilitation program consists of different phases.

2.3.1 Rehabilitation in the acute phase

It covers the first 2 weeks after a stroke and it must be started soon when they are still in the stroke unit [25, 27]. All patients with acute stroke should be evaluated by the rehabilitation physician in the first 24–48 h to assess the deficit and initiate measures to prevent future complications, grade of recommendation A [27].

It is necessary to correctly align the patient in bed, make frequent postural changes, and place the joints in a functional position, with the help of orthoses and pillows. Adduction and internal rotation of the shoulder and flexion of the wrist and hands, as well as hips, knees, and ankles, which tend to extension and varus should be avoided [27].

The immobilization of the muscles in a shortened position is the initial mechanism for the development of contractures, which are objectified as an increase in resistance to passive movement, a situation that, if maintained, will decrease the joint range [26].

Therefore, once the patient is hemodynamically stable, passive kinesitherapy of the affected hemi body will be started [27], performing passive exercises of the full joint arch on a daily basis in the routes susceptible to muscle shortening. Prolonged muscle stretching is more effective than a brief passive exercise. It is also necessary to stimulate the mobility of the unaffected side since immobility weakens its strength [26].

Likewise, the patient will receive instruction to perform functional tasks, such as getting up in the bed and recovering adequate trunk control, which later allows sitting, self-mobilization, and transfers, as well as standing and walking depending on the degree of involvement [27].

In addition, respiratory physiotherapy treatment and global stimulation of the patient should be started [25].

Early mobilization and immediate rehabilitation appear to be the main variables associated with getting the best results in stroke units, by reducing bed-ridden complications (such as aspiration pneumonia, deep vein thrombosis, and pulmonary embolism as a consequence of immobility, contractures and pressure ulcers, potentially avoidable through frequent postural changes) [26].

Current evidence confirms that the more intensive the stroke rehabilitation treatment after the first 24 h, the better the functional results [27].

2.3.2 Rehabilitation in the subacute phase

From 2 weeks to 4 months after the stroke. Patients should be treated both during their hospital stay and after discharge, by units that are specialized in stroke rehabilitation treatment, recommendation grade A [27].

The objective during this phase is to gain the maximum degree of functionality possible by adapting to the deficits [25]. Recovery of motor activity usually follows a proximal to distal order. In cases of partial motor recovery, synergistic mobility patterns may develop. Proximal muscle contraction may induce distal contraction with the mass movement of the limb. The predominant synergies are antigravity: flexor in the upper limb and extensor in the lower [26].

The patient will learn new motor skills through experience and training for the phenomenon that constitutes brain plasticity. This brain reorganization substrate can be modulated by different rehabilitation therapies [26]. These therapies are very varied, and each physiotherapist applies them according to their knowledge and experience. There is no evidence that any type of physiotherapy shows superior results to the others [25].

2.3.2.1 Compensation techniques

They seek to reeducate residual capacities, especially of the unaffected hemi body, to improve function [26]. They are indicated in severe patients with a poor prognosis or in the stabilization phase [25].

2.3.2.2 Neuromotor techniques or facilitating techniques

Their objective is to improve the quality of movement on the affected side. There are different methods [26, 27]:

Bobath method: inhibition techniques (which reduce spasticity, synergies, and abnormal patterns), facilitation techniques (favor the development of normal posture patterns) are applied and the incorporation of the plegic side in therapeutic activities is promoted [25].

Brunnstrom method: It is based on the stimulation of synergies for the performance of analytical movements that the patient does not perform voluntarily [26].

Proprioceptive neuromuscular facilitation (Kabat): its main objective is to improve muscle weakness. It uses peripheral stimuli of superficial (touch) or deep origin (joint position, stretching) to improve muscle strength and coordination. It is based on movement patterns in which weak muscles are aided by stronger agonists [25].

2.3.2.3 Motor relearning techniques or task-oriented rehabilitation

It aimed at improving the execution of specific tasks that have a practical meaning in the patient's life [27]. Learning requires repetitive and intense training, progressive in its difficulty, with feedback on what is being done and motivation strategies [26].

2.3.2.4 Therapy of movement induced by restraint of the healthy side

It is based on experimental studies carried out by Taub in 1977 with monkeys that had undergone a dorsal rhizotomy, showing that they were able to use the affected limb by immobilizing the healthy side [27].

2.3.2.5 Technology applied to task-oriented rehabilitation programs

For example, functional electrical stimulation (FES) applied to the lower extremity as an alternative to an antiequine orthosis or biofeedback to the patient (FES-EMG). Technology can facilitate the automation of the activity to be trained [26].

In this phase, the assessment and treatment of spasticity are also important, and the prescription of drugs or the application of botulinum toxin on the spastic muscles and/or orthoses that maintain muscle stretching may be necessary [25].

Rehabilitative treatment of the upper extremity: Unlike the lower limb, only a minority of patients achieve satisfactory functional use of the upper limb. The purpose of the rehabilitation treatment will be to reach the maximum possible functionality of the affected upper limb [25]. The specific techniques used for its treatment are [27]:

Assisted passive and active kinesitherapy of the affected upper limb, as well as muscle strengthening.

Mental imagery: Mental practice of movements and activities helps the functional recovery of the affected side.

Induced movement therapy with suppression of the healthy side: The best results with this therapy have been obtained when applied 3–9 months after cerebrovascular disease and it has been shown to be superior to conventional therapies in the motor recovery of the paretic upper limb, improving grip and speed of movement in carrying out activities of daily living.

Mirror therapy: It is effective in the motor recovery of the affected limb as well as in the reduction of pain. Visual feedback is used through a mirror, mobilizing both extremities, but observing the healthy side reflected.

Virtual reality: A simulation of the real environment is produced, generating human-computer feedback, while the patient performs the programmed exercises. Currently, it has been shown to be superior to conventional occupational therapy in improving the disability of the affected limb, also enhancing the effects of the latter.

Functional electrical stimulation and simultaneous performance of task-oriented exercises:The synchronization between the increase in sensory inputs to the CNS and muscle contraction stimulates motor recovery.

Robot-assisted therapy in the upper limb: It is used when the patient lacks sufficient strength. As an adjuvant therapy to physiotherapy, it makes it possible to increase the intensity of treatment, improving motor function in the shoulder, elbow and wrist, although it has not been shown to improve ADL performance.

Transcranial stimulation: It favors neuroplasticity phenomena, interfering with the patient's learning and motor function in a noninvasive and safe way.

Rehabilitative treatment of the lower extremity: It should start in the first days. A good mastery of orthostasis and some motor coordination should be achieved as soon as possible [25]. The main objective is to improve mobility and restore motor control of standing and walking (recommendation grade A) [26], to achieve greater independence and reduce energy costs [25]. In general, patients who are capable of performing transfers and standing safely in the subacute phase recover ambulation, in some cases requiring the use of technical aids such as anti-equine orthoses, canes, or a walker [26].

Normally the following phases are followed: initiation of standing, balance re-education, parallel standing, and walking [25]. The following techniques are used [27]:

Passive, assisted and active kinesitherapy, as well as muscle strength training, being the strength of the quadriceps essential for dynamic stability during the support phase of walking.

Re-education of balance: Affected in patients with stroke due to impaired motor control in the trunk and lower extremity, as well as the sensitivity of the corresponding hemibody and a perception disorder, which makes it difficult for the patient to achieve correct maintenance of balance. Its treatment is essential since it can reduce the risk of falls.

Physical reconditioning: It is necessary to carry out an individualized aerobic training program that involves large muscle groups, to combat fatigue and increase cardiovascular resistance. Monitoring of heart rate and blood pressure is recommended during the performance of the same.

Treadmill gait training with or without body weight offloading: It improves gait parameters, increasing monopodal support on the affected side and step alternation, as well as physiological activation of the spinal erectors [25].

FES of the affected lower limb: It improves strength and deformity, but the effect is not maintained over time [25].

Mental imagery [26].

Virtual reality [26].

2.3.3 Rehabilitation in the chronic phase

Rehabilitation is a time-limited process. Beyond the sixth month after the stroke, there is a stabilization phase in functional recovery. To indicate additional intervention in the chronic phase, it is necessary to set a realistic goal, have a rehabilitation technique with evidence of being effective in achieving that goal, and objectify progress towards the planned goal on a practical scale [26].

There are different studies about motor limb rehabilitation.

The AMOBES trial [28] found that additional physical therapy aimed at reducing complications of immobility had similar benefits at a lower dose of physical therapy. Studies performed in the early subacute stage of stroke, treating patients with neuromuscular electrical stimulation, functional stretch training, and task-oriented training, showed similar benefits to routine care for upper extremity functional capacity [29].

The EXPLICIT trial [30] found that restricted movement therapy led to an increase in upper limb capacity in the first 12 weeks after stroke, without maintaining this benefit at 26 weeks.

The VIRTUES [31] and EVREST [32] studies carried out an investigation on the effects of virtual reality and video games on the motor capacity of the upper extremities during the subacute stage of stroke.

The RATULS trial [33] investigated the effects of robot-assisted therapy on upper limb motor ability in the chronic stage of stroke. All of these trials illustrate the feasibility of using these technologies on a large scale and report benefits similar to those produced by an equivalent dose of recreational activities or conventional therapies [29].

2.4 Aphasia and apraxia rehabilitation

Aphasia is an alteration of oral (comprehension and/or expression) or written (reading/writing) language as a consequence of a brain injury. 21–38% of stroke patients will present with some type of aphasia.

Dysarthria is the alteration that occurs in speech as a consequence of muscular dyscontrol in the buccophonatory organs due to the lesion, affecting its clarity.

It is necessary to differentiate it from apraxia, which is the decrease in the ability to voluntarily plan and execute the appropriate movements for the articulation of speech, without affecting the muscles involved in speech [34].

In the subacute and chronic phases, recovery from language and speech disabilities will depend on neuroplasticity processes, so specific assessment by specialized professionals and the start of speech therapy treatment during the subacute phase will be essential [27].

The period of recovery is variable, it is considered that during the first 6 months the speed of recovery is much higher and later it slows down, until almost stabilizing after the first year [26].

The treatment of these patients aims to increase the patient's linguistic capacity, providing them with tools to deal with the situation and make up for the deficit. It should be individualized, early (as soon as the patient is stable, able to cooperate with an acceptable level of care, and not excessively fatigued), and intensive [34]. There is an inverse relationship between the time elapsed from the onset of the deficit to the start of treatment and the magnitude of its effect. The magnitude of the effect is directly related to the frequency and intensity of treatment. The therapies usually offered in our environment, which are usually 2 h/week in the best of cases, have effects that are barely superior to those of spontaneous recovery [27]. Its efficacy has been demonstrated with RCTs with frequencies of 3 h/week or 5 h/week [26].

The speech therapist can opt for three treatment strategies, not mutually exclusive, and that depends on the severity, the evolutionary moment, and the characteristics of each patient [26]:

2.4.1 Recovery of specific linguistic deficits

Recovering the norm, the function is recovered. For example, in Wernicke's aphasia, working on phonological discrimination with specific exercises to differentiate phonemes [26].

2.4.2 Reorganization of the function

Starting from the intact skills. It would be applied to the same patient trying to improve oral comprehension by promoting the use of more preserved semantic comprehension. The important thing is that he understands the messages, not that he maintains certain linguistic skills. It is usually the most used and effective strategy, especially in moderate or severe aphasia [26].

2.4.3 Substitution of lost linguistic abilities by any other mechanism that ensures communication

In the same patient, his or her close environment is taught to increase expressiveness and to increase the gestural code used. It is usually necessary for patients with global or very severe aphasia, in addition to technical aids and augmentative or alternative communication [26].

As long as identifiable goals exist and progress persists, the aphasic patient should continue to receive treatment with regular and objective assessment of progress [25].

2.5 Cognitive and perceptual rehabilitation

Cognitive impairment secondary to stroke is a frequent complication, with a prevalence ranging between 20 and 80%. The risk of cognitive impairment is related to demographic factors (age, education, or occupation of the patient) and vascular factors, although it can be stated in general terms that this risk is increased between 5 and 8 times more after suffering a stroke [35, 36]. Its presence is associated with a lower quality of life 12 months after the stroke, an increased risk of dementia (vascular dementia), mortality and institutionalization rates, as well as an augmented burden on the caregiver and bigger health expenses [37]. However, despite being a common and serious complication that carries a poor prognosis in the medium and long term, it is an underdiagnosed entity [38]. Assessment of cognitive functions should always be done routinely in the clinical care of stroke patients prior to discharge home [39]. To reduce cognitive consequences after stroke, the cognitive impairment must be properly characterized, the underlying causes of cognitive decline understood, and the efficacy of different treatment and rehabilitation approaches determined [40].

Cognition is an aggregate of different cognitive domains that are not independent of each other but are interrelated through neural networks. These cognitive domains could be outlined as follows [40]: attention (focusing, shifting, dividing, or maintaining attention on a particular stimulus or task); executive functions (work planning, organization of thoughts, capacity for inhibition, control, and monitoring of responses, instrumental adaptation); visuospatial skills (visual search, drawing, construction); praxic function and perceptual/recognition skills (gnosis); memory (recall and recognition of visual and verbal information) and language (expressive and receptive, verbal and non-verbal, reading and writing).

A common finding in patients with cognitive impairment secondary to cerebrovascular lesions, and one that appears to be a consistent pattern, it is deficits in attention, executive functions, and processing speed [41]. Memory impairment, highly compromised in patients with Alzheimer's Disease, is not usually the most obvious cognitive deficit after a stroke; only about half of the people with vascular cognitive impairment present amnesic signs, and approximately 30% of patients with vascular cognitive impairment will progress to a phase of dementia [42].

The location of the lesion constitutes a determining factor in the clinic of cognitive deterioration after stroke [43]. Strategic infarcts in specific locations in the brain are capable of causing a postictal cognitive deficit, sometimes of acute/subacute onset. The first evidence in this regard was obtained after observing symptoms of cognitive impairment in the context of acute vascular thalamic lesions.

Some typical locations of strategic infarcts and their most characteristic clinical manifestations are described below (**Table 2**) [44].

The most widely recognized neuropathological substrates include infarcts, hemorrhages, and global hypoxic-ischemic brain injury. White matter injury, including demyelination with or without axonal loss, is also common in people with vascular dementia, but is nonspecific and can also occur in the setting of neurodegenerative dementia, such as in AD. Similarly, cortical atrophy and hippocampal sclerosis may be related to both focal and diffuse hypoxic brain injury, but are also not specific to VD, and are also seen in neurodegenerative diseases [41].

Cognitive rehabilitation plays a fundamental role in multidisciplinary stroke rehabilitation and should be started as soon as possible in order to obtain the best functional results. It should not be done in isolation, but rather combined with physical measures and training in activities of daily living. Furthermore, physical activity by itself protects against cognitive decline by increasing cerebral blood flow and the expression of neurotrophic factors [45]. Interventions carried out in cognitive rehabilitation are broadly classified as direct repair/cognitive skills training to restore previously learned behavior patterns and training of compensatory strategies establishing new patterns of cognitive activity through internal compensatory cognitive

Internal capsule	Frontal lobe dysfunction: inattention, fluctuating alertness, apathy, abulia and psychomotor retardation, memory impairment
Thalamus	Memory impairment, dysexecutive, speed of attention, and mental processing
Fornix	Severe anterograde memory impairment
Caudate Nucleus	Pronounced abulia, disinhibition, and affective disorders
Corpus Callosum	Pure alexia, visual agnosia, unilateral apraxia

Table 2.
Cognitive disorders after strategic strokes.

mechanisms, or establishing new patterns of activity through external compensatory mechanisms such as external aids, environmental structuring, and support [45].

The objectives of cognitive rehabilitation are to reinforce previously learned behavior patterns, establish new patterns of cognitive activity through internal compensatory cognitive mechanisms for impaired neurological systems, establish new patterns of activity through external compensatory mechanisms such as external aid, or structuring and environmental support and to allow people to adapt to their cognitive disability [45].

2.5.1 Rehabilitation in attention, working memory, and processing speed

Rehabilitation in attention, working memory, and processing speed are three cognitive domains that constitute the cognitive triad that must be addressed first for the rehabilitation to be successful. Most exercises are based on the stimulus–response paradigm. The repeated activation and stimulation of the attentional systems facilitate changes in cognitive capacity, progressively increasing the attentional demand. Transcranial magnetic stimulation over the left dorsolateral prefrontal cortex can improve attention [46, 47].

2.5.2 Memory rehabilitation

In mild memory problems, compensatory strategies may be considered [45]. The use of internal strategies (visual images, semantic organization, and spaced practice) is an option for patients with a high degree of functional independence. Non-electronic external strategies (use of notebooks, wall calendars, notes, to-do lists) will be another valid option in patients with preserved executive functions. In more serious deficits, the use of external compensations through assisted technology (e.g., tablets, laptops) is recommended, as well as specific interventions aimed at facilitating the acquisition of specific skills (e.g., error-free learning). Virtual reality games could improve attention and visuospatial memory, while music therapy improves verbal memory.

2.5.3 Rehabilitation of executive functions

Executive dysfunction is the main component of neurobehavioral disorders in these patients [45]. It causes disruptive behaviors that have a great impact on the autonomy, functional independence, and social interaction of the patient. Intervention in groups constitutes a work tool of great value in these cases. It represents an opportunity to observe and work on cognitive and behavioral functioning and interpersonal interaction. The great variety of frontal symptoms (cognitive and behavioral) and the theoretical complexity of the exercises constitute some obstacles to which the designs of executive functional rehabilitation programs are exposed, which is why it is necessary to use different non-exclusive techniques such as modifications of the environment, restoration techniques, compensatory strategies, and educational interventions.

2.5.4 Dual-task training

Dual-task training requires subjects to perform complex cognitive and motor activities simultaneously, improving the coordination of various tasks. Dual tasks are important for different daily activities, such as walking while having a conversation [46].

2.5.5 Pharmacological treatments

Pharmacological treatments (acetylcholinesterase inhibitors, antidepressants, atomoxetine, methylphenidate, and modafinil) have not been shown to improve cognitive impairment in patients with cognitive impairment secondary to stroke, so their use must always be individualized [45].

2.5.6 Rehabilitation of perceptual and constructive abilities

Cortical perceptual abilities are defined as the ability to organize, process and interpret visual, tactile, or kinesthetic afferent information or both, and the capacity to act appropriately on the information received [47]. Some symptoms in relation to the compromise of perceptual activities are unilateral spatial neglect (the lack of information, response, or orientation to sensory stimuli presented on the contralateral side of the lesion, usually related to right parietal lesions. These patients can ignore food on one side of the plate, or attend only to stimuli on one side of the body) [48] and anosognosia (lack of awareness of the loss of an important bodily function, mainly hemiplegia. It is also more common in right parietal lesions) [49]. The left hemisphere is responsible for modulating arousal and attention in the right visual field, while the right hemisphere controls these processes in the left and right visual fields. Rehabilitative interventions must be implemented repeatedly, training the patient to voluntarily compensate for its deficits: seeking adaptation to the external environment with strategies that do not require the patient to be aware of the deficit [49], modifying behavioral conditions to affect the execution of observable tasks, trying to correct hemineglect without the conscious participation of the patient, or with the top-down strategies, in which the voluntary effort of the patient seeks to reduce or compensate the negligent side, following the indications given by the rehabilitator [50].

2.6 Behavior and psychological rehabilitation

The psychological and behavioral changes due to stroke are in most cases devastating, causing a marked decline in quality of life, which can be improved with neurorehabilitation. Anxiety is common during the first year after stroke, with one in three experiencing it, and it gets significantly less attention compared to other psychological problems after stroke. Anxiety significantly influences the quality of life and could be a predictor of depression [51]. Post-stroke depression occurs in 1 in 3 stroke patients and more than half of all cases are neither diagnosed nor treated. Symptoms usually occur within the first three months after the event [52]. These patients experience sleep disturbances, vegetative symptoms, and social withdrawal. In some patients, depression can be accompanied by suicidal thoughts or tendencies. Irritability is a very common symptom after stroke and a source of a great deal of distress to patients and caretakers [53]. All these psychological and behavioral problems can be tackled with group rehabilitation, psychological therapy, and drugs such as selective serotonin reuptake inhibitors.

There are other techniques that can help in mental health recovery and psychological rehabilitation after strokes, such as yoga and meditation. Both are known to reduce anxiety, fear, anger, stress, and depression in patients and caregivers, promote cardio-respiratory health, and reduce stroke-related risk factors such as carotid atherosclerosis, dyslipidemia, hypertension, diabetes, and coronary artery disease. Also, it was demonstrated that following practice of yoga and meditation made significant improvement in muscle power and range of movements in hemiplegic limbs and some positive effects in the Berg Balance Scale, Timed Movement Battery, and quality of life as assessed with the Stroke Impact Scale [54].

2.7 Rehabilitation technologies and remote rehabilitation

Rehabilitation technologies are defined as 'those whose primary purpose is to maintain or improve an individual's functioning and independence, to facilitate participation and to enhance overall well-being' [54]. Such devices are quite helpful in engaging patient's interests and motivation. A wide range of such applications are available:

2.7.1 Robotic devices and virtual reality

Robotic devices are machines capable of carrying out a series of complex actions automatically. Virtual reality consists of machines that produce interactive simulations to allow users to engage in environments that closely resemble the real world. Both techniques use visual and multisensory stimuli and facilitate joint movements, walking, improving muscle strength and motor function. Electromechanically assisted gait training combined with conventional physiotherapy is more effective than training without these devices [54].

To regain motor function after stroke, rehabilitation robots are increasingly integrated into clinics. The devices fall into two main classes: robots developed to train lost motor function after stroke: therapy devices, and robots designed to compensate for lost skills: assistive devices [55].

2.7.2 Electrical stimulation

Electrical stimulation is one of the most widely used therapy and its reported benefits include spasticity reductions, improvements in range of motion, improved sensation, and reduced pain, but its benefit in stroke rehabilitation has not been adequately demonstrated [54].

Remote rehabilitation is very useful after a stroke. Tele-rehabilitation, also known as e-rehabilitation, is the delivery of rehabilitation services over telecommunication networks and the internet, which provides access to rehabilitation services in a remote area using communication technology, minimizing the problem of living far away from these centers where rehabilitation can be offered.

Wearable sensor technology can also address many of these limitations, being able to offer home-based therapies which can be monitored remotely. Brain-computer interface or brain-machine interface is an upcoming technology in stroke rehabilitation, in which brain signals are recorded through a sensor, transmitted to a computer processor to decode it, and formulate a signal for intended actions with a robotic limb or wheelchair [54].

2.8 Predictive factors of recovery

The factors with the greatest weight in the functional prognosis after a stroke are the initial severity, the functionality before the event, the time between the stroke and the start of rehabilitation, and the cognitive status. The two most important predictors of functional recovery are initial stroke severity and age.

The patients who benefit the most from a rehabilitation program are usually those with better baseline functionality. Classification of patients can be made based on the severity of the stroke [8, 10].

2.8.1 Mild stroke

Mild deficits: FIM score > 80. NIHSS <5. There are no assessable cognitive deficits. Barthel >80.

2.8.2 Moderate stroke

Moderate deficits: FIM score 40–80. FIM engine 38–62. NIHSS 5–9. Normal level of consciousness with significant hemiparesis. Barthel 60–80.

2.8.3 Severe stroke

Severe deficits: FIM < 40 or motor FIM < 37. NIHSS >9. It is usually associated with severe motor deficits, impaired level of consciousness, and/or medical comorbidities. Barthel <60.

2.9 Community reintegration

Hospital discharge should never lead to an interruption in rehabilitation, and it is the responsibility of the healthcare organization and the professionals of the rehabilitation teams to ensure the continuity of the process. Hospital discharge planning should be approached from the initial stages of admission and should involve the professionals, the patients themselves, and their families or caregivers. Knowing possible problems and needs in advance facilitates reintegration into the community [51].

The perception of health among people with stroke sequelae 2 years after the stroke is lower than the general population. The factors that determine a lower quality of life are depression, having to depend on a third person, and the need for social help.

Rehabilitation programs are most effective when carried out at an early stage. Late rehabilitation is the one performed when most of the deficits have stabilized and the objective is to maintain recovered functionality, continue the adaptation process, and improve the performance of basic activities of daily life [51].

In patients undergoing rehabilitation programs, improvements in deficits, social participation, and quality of life can be seen even years after the event that generated the initial injury. It is important to make a selection of the appropriate approach to continue the rehabilitation treatment according to the type of patient [9].

2.9.1 Long term care facilities

Patients who continue to need hospitalization and have a moderate or severe disability in more than two functional areas such as mobility, swallowing, or communication, but whose medical and cognitive conditions do not allow them to participate in therapies of high intensity, and without sufficient social and family support to foresee a return home in the medium term.

2.9.2 Outpatient rehabilitation

If patients have a mild or moderate disability and meet the medical and cognitive conditions that allow them to travel to a rehabilitation center, and have good social and family support, they will continue with high-intensity treatment (1–3 h daily) in outpatient rehabilitation centers or by going to the referral hospital on an outpatient basis.

2.9.3 Home rehabilitation

In those patients who continue with a moderate or severe disability and good cognitive conditions but whose medical or social situation does not allow them to travel to a rehabilitation center. For patients with very severe disabilities in the chronic phase, as long as there are functional objectives to be achieved, home rehabilitation can help to avoid long-term complications, readmissions and moderate the impact of the disability on the quality of life of patients and caregivers.

Regarding social support after the stroke, it will be necessary to report on aspects such as labor reintegration, changes, and strategies to minimize sexual dysfunction, the possibility of driving vehicles again, or the access to adapted transport systems that would make it possible to increase the level of occupational, social and leisure activities, improving the quality of life of the patients. In addition, after a stroke, family training and emotional support are highly important, especially for those who are going to become caregivers [51].

Conflict of interest

The authors declare no conflict of interest.

Author details

Iria Beltrán-Rodríguez[1*], Laura García-Talavera Casado[2], Óscar Durán-Borrella[1], Patricia González-Feito[1], Irene Sánchez-Serrano[1] and Rebeca de la Fuente Blanco[1]

1 Complejo Asistencial Universitario de León, León, Spain

2 St. Vincent's University Hospital, Dublin, Ireland

*Address all correspondence to: iriabeltranrodriguez@gmail.com

References

[1] GBD 2016 Neurology Collaborators. Global, regional, and national burden of neurological disorders, 1990-2016: A systematic analysis for the Global Burden of Disease Study 2016. The Lancet. Neurology. 2019;**18**(5):459-480

[2] White H, Boden-Albala B, Wang C, Elkind MS, Rundek T, Wright CB, et al. Ischemic stroke subtype incidence among whites, blacks, and Hispanics: The northern Manhattan study. Circulation. 2005;**111**(10):1327-1331

[3] Schneider AT, Kissela B, Woo D, Kleindorfer D, Alwell K, Miller R, et al. Ischemic stroke subtypes: A population-based study of incidence rates among blacks and whites. Stroke. 2004;**35**(7): 1552-1556

[4] Kleindorfer DO, Khoury J, Moomaw CJ, Alwell K, Woo D, Flaherty ML, et al. Stroke incidence is decreasing in whites but not in blacks: A population-based estimate of temporal trends in stroke incidence from the greater Cincinnati/northern Kentucky Stroke study. Stroke. 2010;**41**(7):1326-1331

[5] Béjot Y, Bailly H, Durier J, Giroud M. Epidemiology of stroke in Europe and trends for the 21st century. Presse Médicale. 2016;**45**(12 Pt 2):e391-e398

[6] Stinear CM, Smith MC, Byblow WD. Prediction tools for Stroke Rehabilitation. Stroke. 2019;**50**(11):3314-3322

[7] Sánchez IE, Martín ME, Izquierdo M. Rehabilitación del Ictus cerebral. En: Sánchez I, Ferrero A, Aguilar J, Climent JM, Conejero JA, Flores MT, et al. Manual SERMEF de Rehabilitación y Medicina Física. Madrid: Panamericana; 2006. p. 479-493

[8] David H, Florencio J, María JV. Manual básicos para residentes medicina fisica y rehabilitacion [Internet]. Maryland Heights, Missouri, United States: Mosby; 1998. ISBN: 978-84-17524-33-3

[9] Francisco M, Miguel Ángel R, Miguel G, María N, Jesús S. Manual de rehabilitación y medicina física [Internet]. Amsterdam, Netherlands: Elsevier; 2002. ISBN: 978-84-09-00977-0

[10] Teasell R, Hussein N. Brain Reorganization, Recovery and Organized Care. Stroke rehabilitation clinician Handbook [Internet]. London, Ontario, Canada: Heart and Stroke Foundation. Canadian Partnership For Stroke Recoverty; 2020. Available from: http://www.ebrsr.com

[11] Muoio V, Persson PB, Sendeski MM. The neurovascular unit—Concept review. Acta Physiologica (Oxford, England). 2014;**210**(4):790-798

[12] Moskowitz MA, Lo EH, Iadecola C. The science of stroke: Mechanisms in search of treatments [published correction appears in Neuron. 2010. Oct 6;68(1):161]. Neuron. 2010;**67**(2):181-198

[13] Doussoulin-Sanhueza MA. Como se fundamenta la neurrorehabilitación desde el punto de vista de la neuroplasticidad. Archivos de Neurociencias (MEX). 2011;**16**(4):216-222

[14] Castillo J. Luces y sombras de la neuroprotección en la isquemia cerebral. Revista de Neuro-Psiquiatria [Internet]. 10 mar. 2013;64(4):354-381

[15] Pozas E. Bases fisiopatológicas de la recuperación tas la isquemia:

neuroplasticidad, neurogénesis y neurorrepatación. En: Montaner-Villalonga, J, coordinador. Neuroreparación y rehabilitación tras el ictus. 1ª. ed. Barcelona: Marge Médica Books; 2010. p. 13-28

[16] Faralli A, Bigoni M, Mauro A, Rossi F, Carulli D. Noninvasive strategies to promote functional recovery after stroke. Neural Plasticity. 2013;**2013**:854597

[17] Hernández S et al. Plasticidad neuronal funcional. Revista de neurología. 2004;**38**(supl. 1):58-68

[18] Laso-Guzmán FJ. Patología del sistema nervioso. En: Laso-Guzmán FJ, editor. Introducción a la medicina clínica. 2ª. ed. Barcelona: Elsevier Masson; 2010. p. 525

[19] Garcés-Vieira MV, Suárez-Escudero JC. Neuroplasticidad: aspectos bioquímicos y neurofisiológicos. Revistas CES Medicina. 2014;**28**(1):119-132

[20] Kreisel SH, Bazner H, Hennerici MG. Pathophysiology of stroke rehabilitation: Temporal aspects of neuro-functional recovery. Cerebrovascular Diseases. 2006;**21**(1-2):6-17

[21] Mahoney FI, Barthel D. Functional evaluation: The Barthel index. Maryland State Medical Journal. 1965;**14**:56-61

[22] Nasreddine ZS, Phillips NA, Bédirian V, Charbonneau S, Whitehead V, Collin I, et al. The Montreal Cognitive Assessment, MoCA: A brief screening tool for mild cognitive impairment. Journal of the American Geriatrics Society. Apr 2005;**53**(4):695-699

[23] Moreno, J.M. y García-Baamonde, Mª.E. Guía de Recursos para la Evaluación del Lenguaje. Madrid: CCS. 2003

[24] Burn JP. Reliability of the modified Rankin scale. Stroke. 1992;**23**(3):438

[25] Fuster A, Morante JL, Ramírez A. Rehabilitación Del Accidente Cerebrovascular. En Alcázar F. Rehabilitación Médica. Aula Médica; 2004

[26] Sánchez I, Martín ME, Izquierdo M. Rehabilitación del Ictus Cerebral. Panamericana: Manual Sermef de Rehabilitación y Medicina Física; 2006

[27] Déniz A, López JC. Enfermedad Cerebrovascular o Ictus: Concepto, Fisiopatología y Evaluación. Tratamiento Rehabilitador. In: Manual de Rehabilitación y Medicina Física. Milan, Italy: Sociedad Canaria de Rehabilitación y Medicina Física; 2018

[28] Yelnik AP, Quintaine V, Andriantsifanetra C, Wannepain M, Reiner P, Marnef H, et al. AMOBES (active mobility very early after Stroke): A randomized controlled trial. Stroke. 2017;**48**(2):400-405

[29] Stinear CM, Lang CE, Zeiler S, Byblow WD. Advances and challenges in stroke rehabilitation. The Lancet Neurology. 2020;**19**(4):348-360

[30] Kwakkel G, Winters C, van Wegen EE, Nijland RH, van Kuijk AA, VisserMeily A, et al. Effects of unilateral upper limb training in two distinct prognostic groups early after Stroke: The EXPLICIT-Stroke randomized clinical trial. Neurorehabilitation and Neural Repair. 2016;**30**(9):804-816

[31] Brunner I, Skouen JS, Hofstad H, Aßmus J, Becker F, Sanders AM, et al. Virtual reality training for upper extremity in subacute Stroke (VIRTUES): A multicenter RCT. Neurology. 2017;**89**(24):2413-2421

[32] Saposnik G, Cohen LG, Mamdani M, Pooyania S, Ploughman M, Cheung D, et al. Efficacy and safety of non-immersive virtual reality exercising in stroke rehabilitation (EVREST): A randomised, multicentre, single-blind, controlled trial. The Lancet. Neurology. 2016;**15**(10):1019-1027

[33] Rodgers H, Bosomworth H, Krebs HI, van Wijck F, Howel D, Wilson N, et al. Robot assisted training for the upper limb after stroke (RATULS): A multicentre randomised controlled trial. Lancet. 2019;**394**(10192):51-62

[34] Peña-Casanova J, Manero RM, Diéguez-Vide F, Sánchez-Benavides G. Afasias. Manual de Logopedia. 4° edición ed. Paris, France: Elvesier, Masson; 2013

[35] Sun JH, Tan L, Yu JT. Post-stroke cognitive impairment: Epidemiology, mechanisms and management. Annals of Translational Medicine. 2014;**2**(8):80

[36] Farokhi-Sisakht F, Farhoudi M, Sadigh-Eteghad S, Mahmoudi J, Mohaddes G. Cognitive Rehabilitation improves ischemic Stroke-induced cognitive impairment: Role of growth factors. Journal of Stroke and Cerebrovascular Diseases. Oct 2019;**28**(10):104299

[37] Donoghue MO, Boland P, Galvin R, Coote S, Hayes S. Rehabilitation of cognitive deficits poststroke: protocol for a systematic review and meta-analysis of randomised controlled trials of non-pharmacological interventions. BMJ Open. 2019;**9**(11):e031052

[38] Godefroy O, Fickl A, Roussel M, Auribault C, Bugnicourt JM, Lamy C, et al. Is the Montreal cognitive assessment superior to the mini-mental state examination to detect poststroke cognitive impairment? A study with neuropsychological evaluation. Stroke. 2011;**42**(6):1712-1716

[39] Winstein CJ, Stein J, Arena R, Bates B, Cherney LR, Cramer SC, et al. Guidelines for adult stroke rehabilitation and recovery: A guideline for healthcare professionals from the American Heart Association/American Stroke Association. Stroke. 2016;**47**(6):e98-e169

[40] Cumming TB, Marshall RS, Lazar RM. Stroke, cognitive deficits, and rehabilitation: Still an incomplete picture. International Journal of Stroke. 2013;**8**(1):38-45

[41] Iadecola C, Duering M, Hachinski V, Joutel A, Pendlebury ST, Schneider JA, et al. Vascular cognitive impairment and dementia: JACC scientific expert panel. Journal of the American College of Cardiology. 2 Jul 2019;**73**(25):3326-3344

[42] Wahlund LO, Erkinjuntti T, Gauthier S. Vascular Cognitive Impairment in Clinical Practice. Cambridge: Cambridge University Press; 2009

[43] Zhao L, Biesbroek JM, Shi L, et al. Strategic infarct location for post-stroke cognitive impairment: A multivariate lesion-symptom mapping study. Journal of Cerebral Blood Flow and Metabolism. 2018;**38**(8):1299-1311

[44] Biesbroek JM, Weaver NA, Biessels GJ. Lesion location and cognitive impact of cerebral small vessel disease. Clinical Science (London, England). 2017;**131**(8):715-728

[45] Alessandro L, Olmos LE, Bonamico L, Muzio DM, Ahumada MH, Russo MJ, et al. Rehabilitación multidisciplinaria Para pacientes adultos con accidente cerebrovascular [multidisciplinary rehabilitation for adult patients with stroke]. Medicina (Buenos Aires). 2020;**80**(1):54-68

[46] Jo JM, Kim YH, Ko MH, Ohn SH, Joen B, Lee KH. Enhancing the working memory of stroke patients using tDCS. American Journal of Physical Medicine & Rehabilitation. 2009;**88**:404-409

[47] Kang EK, Baek MJ, Kim S, Paik NJ. Non-invasive cortical stimulation improves post-stroke attention decline. Restorative Neurology and Neuroscience. 2009;**27**:645-650

[48] Liu KP, Chan CC. Pilot randomized controlled trial of self-regulation in promoting function in acute poststroke patients. Archives of Physical Medicine and Rehabilitation. 2014;**95**(7):1262-1267

[49] Titus MN, Gall NG, Yerxa EJ, Roberson TA, Mack W. Correlation of perceptual performance and activities of daily living in stroke patients. The American Journal of Occupational Therapy. 1991;**45**(5):410-418

[50] Wee JYM, Hopman WM. Comparing consequences of right and left unilateral neglect in a stroke rehabilitation population. American Journal of Physical Medicine and Rehabilitation. 2008;**87**(11):910-920

[51] Rafsten L, Danielsson A, Sunnerhagen KS. Anxiety after stroke: A systematic review and meta-analysis. Journal of Rehabilitation Medicine. 2018;**50**(9):769-778

[52] Llorca GE, Castilla-Guerra L, Moreno MF, Doblado SR, Hernández MJ. Post-stroke depression: An update. Neurología. 2015;**30**(1):23-31

[53] Mimentza N, González-Fraile E, Arango-Lasprilla JC, Ortiz-Marqués N, Berrios GE, González-Pinto A, et al. Assessing irritability in patients with stroke: Psychometric properties of the irritability questionnaire. Brain Injury. 2020;**34**(1):115-121

[54] Sanchetee P. Current trends in stroke rehabilitation. En: Ischemic Stroke. IntechOpen: London; 2021

[55] Klamroth-Marganska A. Stroke rehabilitation: Therapy robots and assistive devices. Advances in Experimental Medicine and Biology. 2018;**1065**:579-587

Chapter 2

Stroke and Healthcare Facilities in Bangladesh and Other Developing Countries

Mohammad Shaikhul Hasan, Kanida Narattharaksha, Md. Sazzad Hossain and Nahar Afrin

Abstract

Globally, healthcare systems are struggling to make a healthier citizen by dropping infectious and non-infectious diseases. South-east Asian countries have achieved several Millennium Development Goals (MDG) with the efforts of better health system management. For instance, in the year 2015, the healthcare system of Bangladesh has achieved the MDG-Four in reducing the infant mortality rate and growth rate. Even then, the life-threatening diseases still remain as a major challenge to the healthcare systems in Bangladesh. Among those, non-communicable diseases (NCDs) are the major cause of death, and stroke is the second leading NCD in accordance with causes of death and long-term disability in Bangladesh. The majority as 80% of stroke survivors are living with either minor or major physical, emotional, and cognitive disabilities. They could get back to their functional life through comprehensive rehabilitation services. Nevertheless, information on the availability of rehabilitation services is not visible to all citizens of Bangladesh. That's why more than half of all stroke survivors are dying on their way to the hospital to seek health care facilities. Therefore, the aim of this literature review was to present a clear vision of the healthcare system and the path of care to all citizens of Bangladesh.

Keywords: post-stroke, rehabilitation, non-communicable diseases (NCDs), Bangladesh healthcare service systems

1. Introduction

Stroke is the leading non-communicable disease worldwide and in the Southeast Asia (SEA) region [1]. In Bangladesh, stroke is the second leading non-communicable disease in terms of the cause of death and long-term disability. Those who survived from stroke attack need quality rehabilitation services to maintain their health and prevent them from death due to the second episode of stroke attack [2]. The quality of services can be viewed from many perspectives. However, the patient perspective is now given more importance because it can lead to the effectiveness of healthcare services and better health outcomes. Therefore, this study aims to examine the level of patient expectations and perceptions and the factors relating to the patient expectations and perceptions of outpatient post-stroke rehabilitation services delivery management in Bangladesh.

This chapter includes an overview of Bangladesh, health status and challenges, stroke definition and situation, post-stroke situation and how Bangladesh healthcare service systems respond to the post-stroke, stroke, and post-stroke care pathway and quality of post-stroke rehabilitation services as well as the methodology to examine the quality of post-stroke rehabilitation services and conceptual framework of this research study.

2. Overview of Bangladesh

Bangladesh is one of the smallest and most densely populated countries in the world. It is a developing country and a founding member of the South Asian Association of Regional Cooperation (SAARC) to promote regional connectivity and cooperation. Additionally, it is a member of the Commonwealth of Nations [3].

2.1 Geography

Bangladesh is a country in the South Asia Region [3]. According to the Ministry of Health and Family Welfare [4], geographically it is divided into eight divisions/provinces, and the total land area of this country is 147,570 sq. km. Dhaka division is the central division, and Dhaka city is the capital city of Bangladesh followed by Rajshahi, Barishal, Chittagong, Sylhet, Mymensingh, Khulna, and Rangpur divisions. Bangladesh National Portal [5] reported that the divisions/provinces are

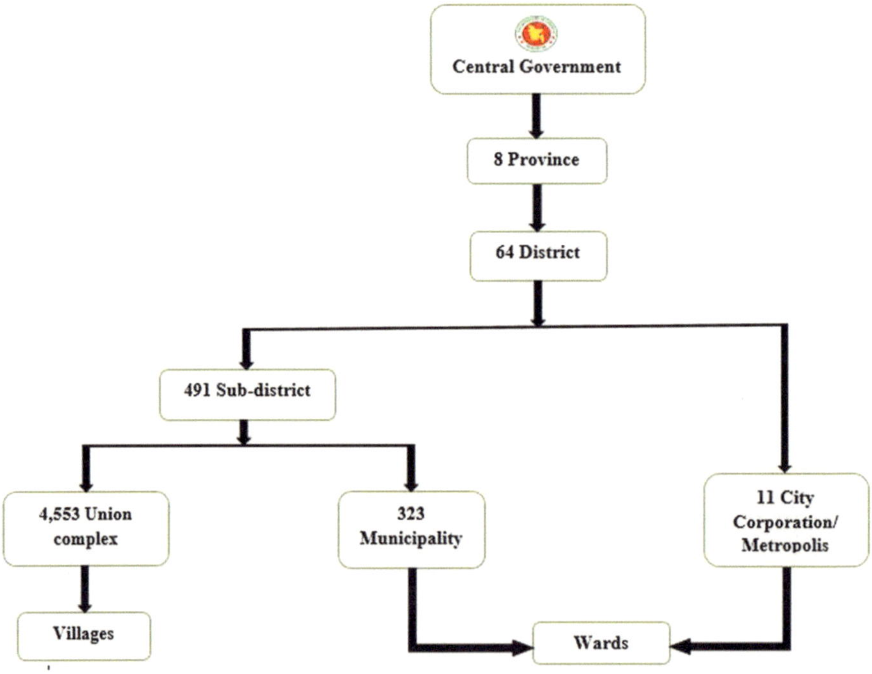

Figure 1.
The administrative geography of the Government of Bangladesh. Adopted from: Bangladesh National Portal [5].

divided into 64 districts and 11 metropolises. Under the districts, there are 491 sub-districts. The sub-districts contain 4553 union councils in the rural areas and 323 municipalities in the urban areas. Consequently, a ward is under the municipality and the municipality is under the metropolis. There is no specific number of wards and villages. **Figure 1** demonstrates the overall administrative geography of the government of Bangladesh.

3. Socio-demographic and economic

The World Bank [6] reported that approximately 162 million people are living in this country. The World Bank [6] also claimed that in 2016, there are nearly 1253 people per sq. km. However, nearly 35% of the total population are living in urban areas for their employment.

The economic status of the citizens is improving, but still, possibly 25% of the total population are living under the poverty line [7]. In the year 2016, the growth domestic product (GDP) per capita was 1358.78 US$, and in the same year, the annual growth rate was 7.11 US$ [6].

4. Health status and challenges

According to Muhammad et al. [8], the healthcare system of Bangladesh has achieved the Millennium Development Goal Four (MDG-4) by reducing infant mortality rate and growth rate, and maternal and child health improvement. Consequently, life expectancy at birth has increased. As an example, the World Bank [9] reported that in 2005, the life expectancy at birth was 67.94 years and in the year 2015, it reached 72.22 years (i.e. male 70.59 years and female 73.94 years). It is comparatively higher than other state members in SAARC. As evidence, the Bhutanese life expectancy was 69.8 years; Indian was 68.3 years, and Myanmar was 66.3 years in the year 2015 data. However, Ahmed et al. [10] claimed that the health system of Bangladesh had achieved MDG-4 and better life expectancy, though several life-threatening diseases still remain.

The top five causes of death in Bangladesh are heart disease, stroke, Chronic Obstetric Pulmonary Diseases (COPD), lower respiratory infections, and diabetes [11]. The mortality rate of infectious diseases, maternal, prenatal, and nutritional conditions gradually went down from 30.9% in the year 2010 to 25.3% of total death in the year 2015 [12]. Relatively, the mortality rate of non-communicable diseases is now rising and going to be a major health challenge and life-threatening diseases in Bangladesh [8]. NCDs caused almost 67% of the total death [9]. Significantly, stroke caused more than half of the total NCD fatalities in Bangladesh [13]. And due to the shortage of the health workforce and inefficient management, it was difficult to provide proper services for people who had strokes [4]. **Table 1** demonstrated all related data by selecting the major geographical, socio-demographic, economic, and health status of the citizens of Bangladesh.

4.1 Stroke definition and situation

According to the American Stroke Association [15], stroke is one of the NCDs which is a medical emergency characterized by a neurological deficit attributed to an

Subject	Indicators	Value
Area	Total land area (sq. km)	147,570
Population	Total population in the year 2016 (in million)	162
	Density in 2016 (per sq. km)	1251.84
	Crude birth rate in 2015 (per 1000)	19.23
	Crude death rate in 2015 (per 1000)	5.31
Life-expectancy	Male in the year 2016 (at birth)	70.59
	Female in the year 2016 (at birth)	73.94
	Total in the year 2016 (at birth)	72.22
Economic condition	GDP per capita in 2016 (US $)	1358.78
	GDP per capita PPP in 2016 (US $)	3580.70
	Annual Growth rate in 2016	7.11
Ethnicity	Muslim (% of total population)	90
	Hinduism (% of total population)	9
	Others (% of total population)	1
Communicable diseases	Total mortality rate in 2015 (% of total death)	25.3
Non-communicable diseases	Total mortality rate in 2015 (% of total death)	66.9

Sources: World Bank [6, 9, 12]; Ahmed et al. [10]; and A. Islam [14].

Table 1.
Major selected geography, socio-demographic, economic, and health status of Bangladesh in the years 2015 and 2016.

acute focal injury of the central nervous system (CNS) by a vascular cause, including cerebral infarction, intracerebral hemorrhage (ICH), and subarachnoid hemorrhage (SAH) and it is a major cause of disability and death worldwide.

Nearly 4.46 million people have died due to stroke per year; 1.2 million in developed countries and nearly 3.2 million in developing countries [16]. For example, stroke was the 4th leading cause of death for US citizens in the year 2010 [17]. In every 40 seconds, someone was attacked by a stroke, and in every 4 minutes, someone died because of the stroke. It was also the leading cause of long-term disability in the United States. Similarly, in the year 2012 Australia projected that 377,000 people had a stroke sometime in their lives; and in 2013, the estimated deaths due to stroke were 8100 people [18]. Additionally, the stroke prevalence in European countries was also more similar to that in other countries. In 2015, it was found that, in the Netherlands, 0.2% of the total population had suffered from stroke each year [19]. Moreover, in 2008, around 3.7 million Southeast Asian people died from stroke. Islam et al. [20] reported that in Bangladesh, approximately 48,951 people had died due to stroke.

According to mortality, morbidity, and long-term disability rate, stroke is the second leading NCD in Bangladesh [11]. Nearly 113.9 persons per 100,000 had died due to stroke in the year 2013, and the increasing rate per year was 4.9% [21]. A total of 20% stroke patients died immediately in the acute phase, and 80% of the stroke survivors lived with minor or major disabilities [22]. Moreover, Centre for Injury Prevention Health Development and Research Bangladesh (CIPRB) [23] reported that approximately 15 out of 1000 Bangladeshi people were affected by stroke. Additionally, Islam et al. [20] found that the prevalence of stroke is 0.03% and it is snowballing. Nearly 485 out of 10,000 people died suffering from stroke disability [20]. Mamin et al. [24] found that nearly 82.5% Bangladeshi stroke survivors' age ranged between 41 and 60 years. Consequently, the big proportions of working people have lost their functional ability and it greatly impacts the economy of Bangladesh.

4.2 Stroke impact

The American Stroke Association [25] claimed that the stroke effects depend on the lesion of the area of the brain cell. Different areas of the brain cell are responsible for different activities. Due to the lesion of the brain cell, the stroke effects can be physical paralysis, memory loss, speech loss, emotional, and behavioral problems. Wolfe [26] claimed that the stroke impacts could be explained from the perspectives of the government, society, family, and patient. From there, the socio-economic impact of stroke is more common in developing countries. Similarly, Institute for Health Metrics and Evaluation [11] reported that a stroke is a great economic burden for a developing country like Bangladesh.

According to Mamin et al. [24], nearly 77% of stroke survivors were public or private or self-employed in Bangladesh. Similarly, Global Health Statistics [21] reported that a big proportion of the working-age group and healthy life had been lost due to stroke in Bangladesh. For example, an estimated 1259.1 people at the age range of 30–34, 9102.9 people at the age range of 50–54, and 21695.5 people at the age range of 60–64 were affected by stroke and lost their functional life in the year 2014. Therefore, the government of Bangladesh has lost a big proportion of its workforce, and it greatly impacts the government and the economy.

Besides, Mohammad [22] claimed that the physical limitation of the patients greatly impacted the patients' participation in the social programs or activities in society. They need long-term hospitalization and rehabilitation services, and the family has to look after them. However, Disability in Bangladesh (2004) reported that it is difficult to bear the whole treatment cost and the health system of Bangladesh has no health insurance package for their citizens. Therefore, it is also an economic burden for their families [11]. According to Mohammad [22], the burden of stroke is not only for their families, but it is also a burden for the patient because of their post-stroke disabilities and impairments.

4.3 Post-stroke

The post-stroke means a group of conditions including physical disability, emotional disturbance, and loss of cognition [27]. At the post-stroke phase, patients suffered from several complications; such as pressure sores, urinary tract infections (UTI), joint contraction, aspiration pneumonia, and recurrent stroke due to lack of proper healthcare services [2]. Consequently, these complications could be a leading reason for readmission and also for excruciating death. Gordon et al. [28] reported that daily activity or daily routine exercise helps the post-stroke patients' to reduce immobility and make them as functional as possible. Therefore, the post-stroke phase is more crucial. Additionally, Runa [29] found that post-stroke complication is a very common problem in Bangladesh.

Accordingly, Mohammad [22] claimed that better care and rehabilitation services could get them back to their independent life. The better quality of healthcare services means a better patient experience, and it is associated with better health outcomes with a higher level of loyalty to follow preventive and treatment strategies of the hospital personnel [30]. Therefore, the healthcare system needs to ensure better and sustainable healthcare services to reduce post-stroke patients' complications by increasing the better patient experience and patient participation in healthcare [31].

4.4 Healthcare service delivery systems

The health system is a dynamic and enduring obligation to peoples' health throughout their lifespan [32]. The primary purpose of the health system is to provide healthcare services to promote, restore or maintain the health of the nation [33]. According to the healthcare policy and *Constitution Act 18* cited in Ministry of Law [34], the fundamental principle of the health system of Bangladesh is to ensure better healthcare services for their citizens. The healthcare system of Bangladesh has been providing a comprehensive healthcare service by following multilevel healthcare service delivery processes [35]. The comprehensive healthcare service includes curative, rehabilitative, promotive, and preventive services. In accordance with service delivery processes, the three levels of health care services are being considered in the health systems of Bangladesh. Such as tertiary, secondary, and primary care levels of healthcare services.

4.5 Tertiary care level

All the national specialized and medical college hospitals are providing the tertiary level of healthcare services [10]. According to the Ministry of Health and Family Welfare [4], there are numerous condition-based specialized hospitals and 14 medical college hospitals that provide the tertiary level of healthcare services, and these are the highest level of referral hospitals in the health system of Bangladesh. Ahmad [36] reported that this tertiary care concentrated more on curative and intensive healthcare services along with rehabilitative care services and ignored the promotive and preventive care services. Besides, Mamin et al. [24] claimed that the public hospitals also wanted to avoid these rehabilitation services in the health systems of Bangladesh.

In regard to stroke care, all public and private hospitals are serving their in-patient intensive curative care and treatment services [4]. However, only a few of them are providing after-stroke rehabilitation services at the physical rehabilitation department on an out-patient basis [37]. Separately, the non-profit organization as the Centre for the Rehabilitation of the Paralyzed (CRP) is providing after-stroke rehabilitation services in both ways (i.e. in-patient and out-patient basis) [38]. The CRP also extended its branches and services across the six divisions in the health systems of Bangladesh [39].

4.6 Secondary care level

According to the Ministry of Health and Family Welfare [4], secondary care or less intensive care is being provided at the district general hospitals. There are 62 district general hospitals to serve their secondary care services throughout the districts of the country. Secondary care includes curative, promotive, and preventive services. The promotive and preventive care services are being provided only for infectious diseases (i.e. Tuberculosis, Malaria, influenza, etc.) [40]. These secondary care hospitals are the first referral hospital in the health system of Bangladesh, and it does not provide rehabilitation services.

4.7 Primary care level

According to the Ministry of Health and Family Welfare [4], primary care includes curative, promotive, and preventive treatment facilities along with rehabilitative services. The primary care services are being provided at the sub-district or Upazila level, union level, and community level. At this primary care level, the public sector provided the services free of charge. The Upazila health complex and Union sub-centers are committed to providing curative, promotive, and preventive services only. There are 491 Upazila health complex hospitals and 3134 Union Sub-centers at the primary care level to provide in-patient and out-patient services. There are 13,336 community clinics serving maternal and child-related outdoor primary care services with basic medicines. Besides, Biswas et al. [40] reported that the Upazila health complex with the cooperation of NGOs has been running an NCD corner (i.e. fast-track corner) at the primary care level of Bangladesh to prevent the risk factors of NCDs. Consequently, due to the lack of healthcare personnel of the public sector, the NGOs are providing community-based rehabilitation services at this primary care level free of charge.

Table 2 lists all the hospitals and other healthcare facilities beneath the Directorate General of Health Services (DGHS) of the Ministry of Health and Family Welfare of Bangladesh. There is no list of private hospitals; thus, only public hospitals' information is listed in the table. In this table, the type of hospital services includes inpatient and outpatient types of services.

4.8 Human resources

The Ministry of Health and Family Welfare [41] reported that there were 74,099 physicians, 6,481 dental surgeons, almost 46,000 registered nurses, 775 pharmacists, 6,029 medical technologists, and 66,623 community health workers. The number of physicians and population ratio was 4.5 per 10,000 populations. There was no more data on the rehabilitation professionals, only a little information available about the physical therapist. The Ministry of Health and Family Welfare [4] reported that in the public sector, nearly 117 physiotherapists are working. Separately, World Confederation for Physical Therapy (WCPT) [42] reported that approximately 1,600 physiotherapists are working in the whole Bangladesh healthcare service sectors. According to a 2016 report of the Bangladesh Health Professionals Institute (BHPI), 241 occupational therapists have graduated and are working in various national and international organizations and hospitals in the country and abroad [43]. The Society of Speech and Language Therapists (SSLTs) reports that speech and language therapy is a relatively new profession in comparing with other rehabilitation professions in Bangladesh and as of 2016, there are 104 graduate speech and language therapists those are working in various national and international healthcare organizations in Bangladesh [44]. Approximately, 25 to 30 students from each department of BHPI (the academic institute of CRP) (Occupational Therapy and Speech and Language Therapy) completing their graduate program each year and initiate clinical practices [39]. **Table 3** demonstrated the healthcare personnel and population ratio of serving healthcare services healthcare services in Bangladesh. Therefore, the availability of rehabilitation services and the fee for the services are the greatest challenge for the person with rehabilitation service needs.

4.9 Financial challenges

According to Bangladesh National Health Accounts [45], the total health expenditure was only 3.5% of the total GDP. It is relatively low, and according to per capita, the health expenditure was 27 US$. However, from this expenditure, the

Level of facilities	Type of facilities	Type of services	Total no. of facilities	Bed occupancy
Secondary & Tertiary level hospitals and other facilities under DGHS				
District	50-bed hospital	Hospital	2	100
	District & General hospital	Hospital	65	10,328
Divisional & National level	Chest diseases hospital	Hospital	13	866
	Dental college hospital	Hospital	1	200
	Hospital for alternative	Hospital	2	200
	medicine	Hospital	5	180
	Infectious disease hospital	Hospital	3	130
	Leprosy hospital	Hospital	14	12,963
	Medical college hospital	Hospital	4	325
	Other hospitals	Hospital	3	850
	Specialized hospital	Hospital	11	3184
	Specialty post-graduate	Hospital	5	100
	institute and hospital	Hospital	1	N/A
	Trauma centre	Hospital	1	N/A
	Chittagong skin & hygiene	Hospital	1	N/A
	treatment centre			
	National asthma centre			
	National centre for control of rheumatoid fever and heart diseases			
Total number of hospitals and other facilities			131	29,426
Primary level healthcare facilities				
Upazila	Upazila health complex (50	Hospital	297	14,850
	bed)	Hospital	113	3503
	Upazila health complex (31	Hospital	11	110
	bed)	Hospital	3	0
	Upazila health complex (10	Outdoor	60	......
	bed)	Hospital	5	155
	Upazila health complex (0	Hospital	2	60
	bed)			
	Upazila health office			
	31-bed hospital			
	30-bed hospital			
Total Upazila level facilities			491	18,678
Union	20-bed hospital	Hospital	32	640
	10-bed hospital	Hospital	19	190
	Union sub-center	Outdoor	1498	......
	Union health and family welfare center	Outdoor	1585	......
Total union level facilities			3134	830
Word	Community clinic (at present)	Outdoor	13,336	......
Grand total primary level hospitals			482	19,508
Grand total primary level facilities			16,968	19,508
Grand total health facilities under DGHS of Bangladesh			17,099	48,934

Source: Ministry of Health and Family Welfare [4].

Table 2.
The hospitals and other healthcare facilities under the DGHS of Bangladesh.

Healthcare providers and population ratio		
Healthcare personnel	**Number**	**Ratio**
Physician	74,099	4.5: 10,000 people
Neurologist	60	0.004: 10,000 people
Dental surgeons	6481	0.40: 10,000 people
Registered nurse	46,000	2.84: 10,000 people
Physical therapist	1600	0.1: 10,000 people
Occupational Therapist	241	0.024: 10,000 people
Speech and Language Therapist	104	0.010: 10,000 People
Community health worker	66,623	4.11: 10,000 people

Source: Ministry of Health and Family Welfare [4, 41], BHPI [43] and SSLTs [44].

Table 3.
The healthcare professional and population ratio in the years 2015 and 2016.

government invested only 23%, and the rest of the amount came from out-of-pocket payments. According to Ahmed et al. [10], this out-of-pocket payment was almost 63% of total healthcare cost. Besides, there was no specific budget for stroke and post-stroke patients and their healthcare services. Moreover, the Ministry of Health and Family Welfare [4] reported that they invested only 2714 million BDT taka (32 million US$) for overall NCDs surveillance. This was a very small expenditure compared to the expenditures on communicable and maternal diseases (i.e. 579 million US$) in the healthcare service system of Bangladesh. Therefore, financial challenge is a big challenge to provide NCD-related healthcare programs in the healthcare system of Bangladesh.

4.10 Policy and programs

Since the liberation, the health system of Bangladesh has been concentrating on controlling communicable and maternal and child-related diseases [10]. Global Health Statistics [21] reported that within the last decade the burden of NCDs is snowballing and has become a major health challenge for Bangladeshi citizens. Furthermore, the Ministry of Health and Family Welfare concentrated on this issue, and with the cooperation of NGOs and private organizations, they developed different policies and had been implementing these to strengthen the healthcare system of Bangladesh [40].

There is no specific policy and program for after stroke disability. All the policies are focused on preventive and promotive health care services to control the risk factors of NCDs including stroke. However, these services are also important to reduce the second episode of stroke attack [46] such as the Health, Nutrition and Population Strategic Investment Plan (HNPSI) for six years (2016–2021) to inter-organization collaborative work and improve healthy lifestyles [4]; *The Smoking and Tobacco Products Usages (control) Act, 2013* to reduce smoking [5]. Furthermore, the governance, non-governance, and private organizations are working collaboratively to implement these policies and programs [40]. One example is the NCDs intervention corner at the primary care level of Bangladesh.

4.11 Governance and organizations

The health system of Bangladesh has been following a pluralistic healthcare system. The Ministry of Health and Family Welfare is the main government organization of the health system of Bangladesh [4]. This ministry is responsible for providing curative, promotive, and preventive services through tertiary care, secondary care, and primary care organizations. For rehabilitation services, the Ministry of Social Welfare is the responsible government organization, but at present both ministries (i.e. Ministry of Health and Family Welfare and Ministry of Social Welfare) are working collaboratively to serve rehabilitation services at the different levels of healthcare services [47].

The public sector in the health systems of Bangladesh did not concentrate more on rehabilitation services [24]. Thus, the private sectors (for-profit organizations) and NGOs (not-for-profit organizations) extended their healthcare services including rehabilitation services [20]. A few of the private hospitals are providing post-stroke rehabilitation services at tertiary care level hospitals on an inpatient and outpatient basis.

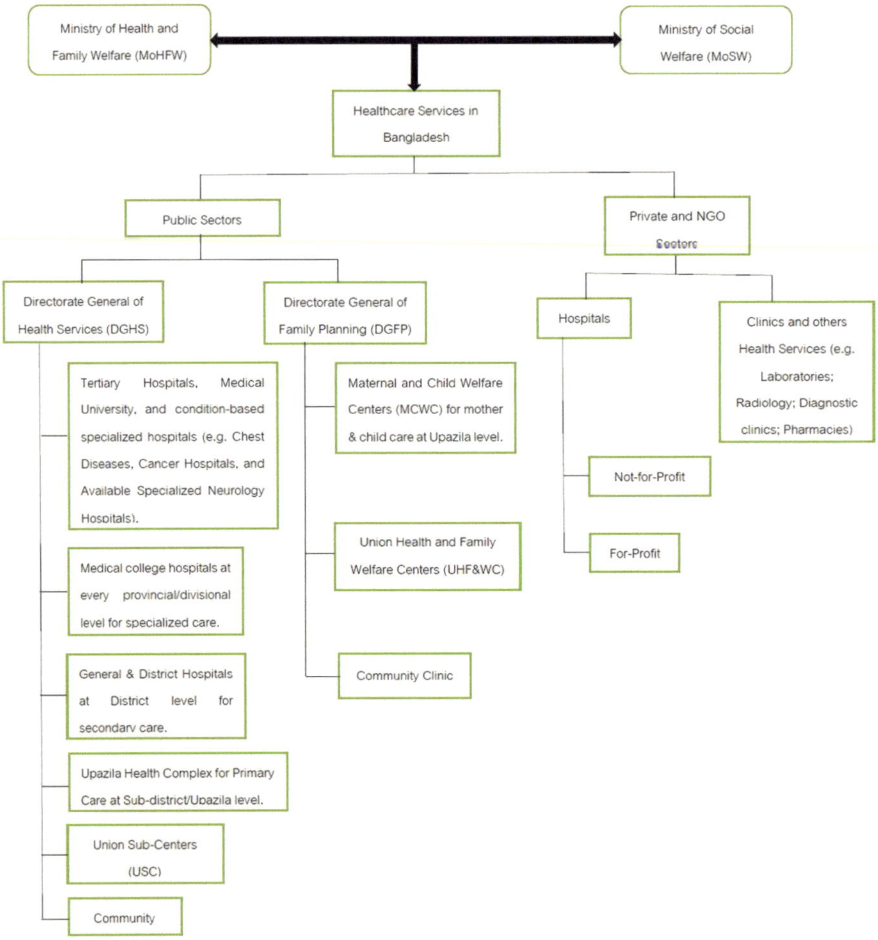

Figure 2.
Health service systems structure in Bangladesh health systems. Adopted from: Ministry of Health and Family Welfare [4]; Ahmed et al. [10]; Biswas et al. [40].

Along with the private sectors, several NGOs under the Ministry of Social Welfare have been offering post-stroke rehabilitation services within the community and hospital [40]. These NGOs are the Bangladesh Rehabilitation Assistance Committee (BRAC), Handicap International (HI), International Committee of the Red Cross (ICRC), and the CRP (Handicap International (HI) [48] and Islam et al. [20]). The International Committee of the Red Cross (ICRC) with the collaboration of CRP has been providing rehabilitation services in the community [49]. While only the CRP provides hospital-based stroke rehabilitation services besides community-based rehabilitation services.

The CRP is offering rehabilitation services throughout the six divisions of the administrative geography of Bangladesh [39]. The CRP is also committed to provide Multi-Disciplinary Team (MDT) based rehabilitation services. According to Gresham et al. [50], the rehabilitation services by a multidisciplinary team provide better health outcomes after-stroke disabilities. The MDT approach consists of different specialists or professionals, those working in a team according to the needs of the patient [51]. In this approach, all professionals are offering their highest potential skills to change the patients' condition as much as possible. **Figure 2** demonstrates the overall service structures of the Bangladesh healthcare system.

5. The Centre for the Rehabilitation of the Paralyzed (CRP)

According to CRP [39], the CRP is a not-for-profit NGO to serve rehabilitation services for person with disabilities. CRP's vision is "to ensure the inclusion of girls and boys, women and men with disabilities into mainstream society." To achieve this vision, CRP worked with several missions such as "to promote an environment where all girls and boys, women and men with disabilities have equal access to health, rehabilitation, education, employment, the physical environment, and information." The CRP is coordinated by a committee, and it is committed to serving quality services.

Trust for Rehabilitation of the Paralyzed (TRP) is the central committee and all the decisions such as policy, programs, and implementation are being addressed by the recommendation of this committee. The executive director coordinates all the CRP services throughout the CRP branches. The program manager helps the executive director to coordinate all the programs. The program manager divides all the CRP activities into various programs or services. Every wing is being coordinated by the head of the wing along with several heads of the departments. Additionally, there is the academic wing to provide the skillful rehabilitation professionals to serve the quality services toward the patients. It has ten branches, and the medical service wing is responsible for serving all healthcare services.

In this context, the physical therapy department is responsible for recovering physical functions, the occupational therapy department for recovering daily activities, and the speech and language therapy department for recovering communication and swallowing difficulties. According to CRP policy, all medical professionals have to wear hospital uniform during therapy services. Only the five CRP divisional hospital branches (i.e. Rajshahi, Chittagong, Barisal, Sylhet- Moulvibazar, and Mymensingh branches) along with the main branch of Dhaka division has been providing the out-patient medical services and rehabilitation services. The rest of the branches are responsible for providing Community-Based Rehabilitation (CBR) services and health promotion and prevention activities beneath the rehabilitation wing. CBR is offering these services five full days a week, from 8 am to 5 pm.

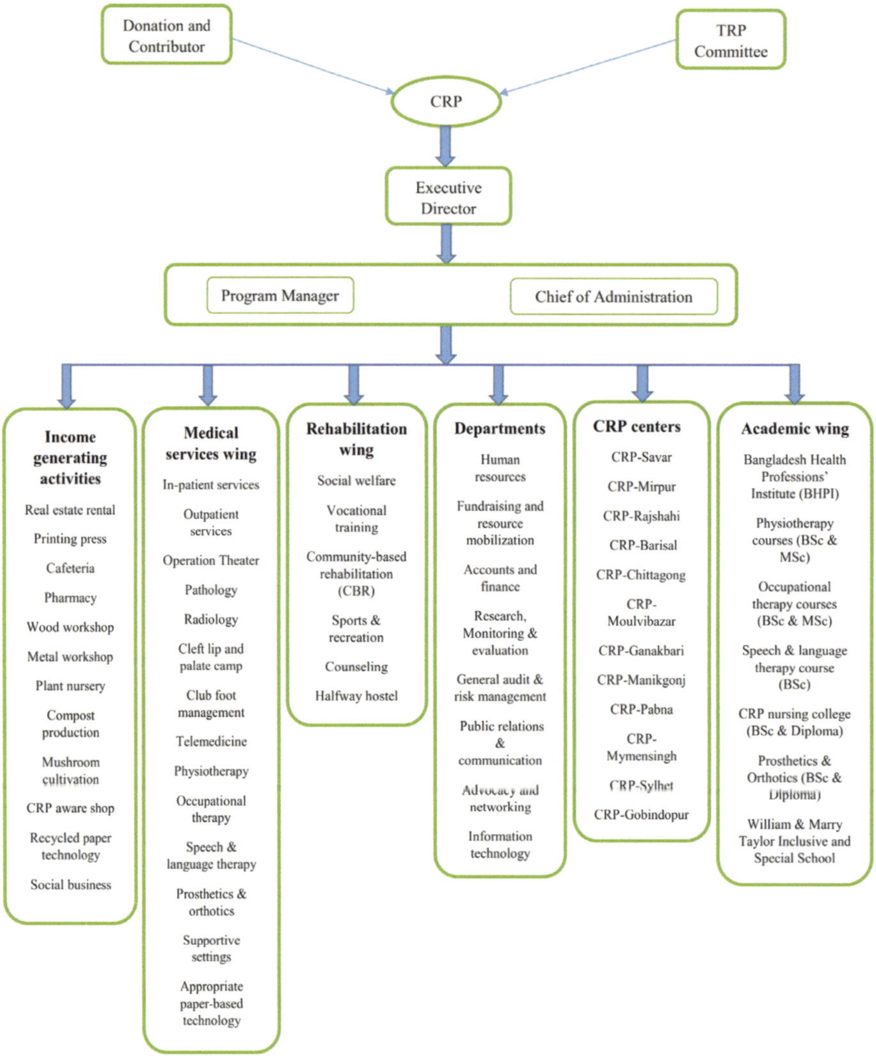

Figure 3.
The organogram of the CRP activities in Bangladesh. Sources: Adapted from [39].

There are several departments, and the research and evaluation department coordinates all the research-oriented formalities in the CRP. CBR collects donation and undergoes several income-generating activities to enhance the endowment to run the healthcare services (i.e. CRP cafeteria, nursery, woodshop, etc.). **Figure 3** demonstrates the CRP management organogram with several services and activities throughout the country.

6. The rehabilitation personnel in the CRP hospital

The CRP (2016) reported that all of 755 dedicated employees are working throughout this organization and its branches. However, there is no exact data for the total number of separate rehabilitation professionals.

7. Stroke and post-stroke care pathways in Bangladesh

The rehabilitation service systems and stroke care depend on the severity of the patients and the episodes of the stroke attack [52]. They have mentioned two phases; the acute phase and the sub-acute phase of stroke care. However, Pitthayapong et al. [2] added the post-stroke phase and it is started at the end of the acute and subacute periods of stroke.

7.1 Acute stroke care

Acute stroke care means care that takes place 24–48 hours after stroke, and during this period they need more intensive comprehensive services including rehabilitation if possible [52]. Particularly, inpatient rehabilitation care units of the hospitals serve the acute stroke care services, and the tertiary/specialized hospitals and divisional general hospitals provide comprehensive stroke care services under the healthcare services structure of Bangladesh (Directorate General of Health Services [53]; Bhowmik et al. [7]; & Nessa et al. [37]).

7.2 Subacute stroke care

At the end of the acute period of stroke, the sub-acute period of stroke starts, and the duration of this phase is one week until one month [52]. At this period the neurological condition of the stroke patients is more stabilized than during the acute stroke period, and from this phase, they attend a regular rehabilitation program [54]. The acute and sub-acute stroke patient services are similarly available in the tertiary/specialized hospitals and divisional general hospitals in Bangladesh (Directorate General of Health Services [53]; Bhowmik et al. [7]; Nessa et al. [37]).

7.3 Post-stroke care

Post-stroke care is care that started at the end of the acute and sub-acute phase of stroke patients [55]. However, Habib and Hirschfeld [56] found that the post-stroke care with the integration of rehabilitation services was effective. The limited specialized public and private hospitals at the tertiary level and the CRP hospital provide after-stroke/post-stroke rehabilitation services. The NGOs and Upazila health complex hospitals provide preventive and promotive services for reducing the risk factors of the second episode of stroke attack in the health systems of Bangladesh (Biswas et al. [40] & Ahmed et al. [10]).

The stroke care pathways in the Bangladesh health service system are complex and difficult to control. According to Biswas et al. [40], first, the patient visits the Upazila health complex, and if the responsible health professional notices any signs and symptoms of the stroke risk factors, then they suggest that the patient has to continue the preventive and promotive services from the NCDs corner. Directorate General of Health Services [53] reported that according to the stroke management guideline; if the patient needs emergency services, they are referred to the district hospital for secondary care. Thus, the district hospital takes care of this patient according to their available resources. If the patient's condition becomes more severe, then the district hospital refers the patient to the tertiary or specialized hospitals for more intensive care and neurological treatment.

According to this stroke management guideline, after completing the acute stage, some of the hospitals send them to the rehabilitation hospital or the rehabilitation unit of the hospitals for early rehabilitation services [53]. Moreover, the rehabilitation

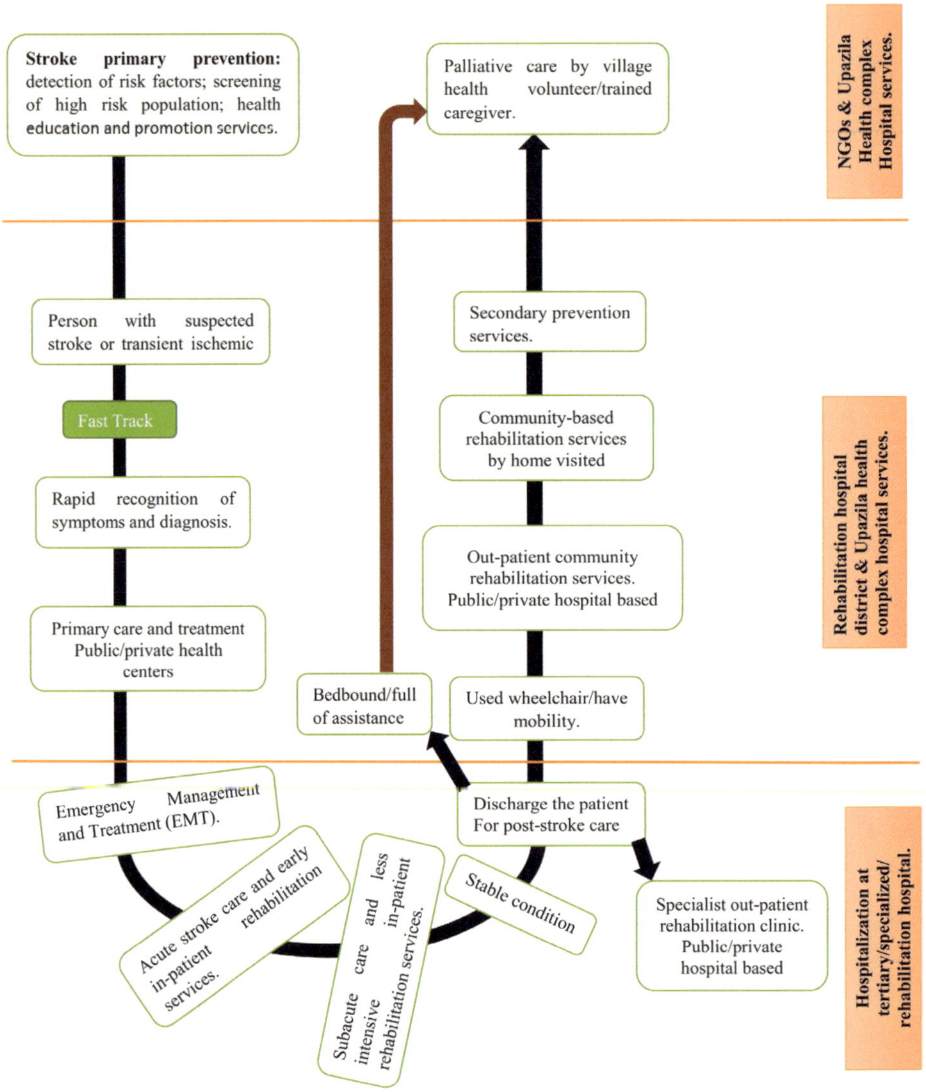

Figure 4.
Stroke and post-stroke care pathways along with the rehabilitation services in Bangladesh. Adopted from: Directorate General of Health Services [53]; Ahmed et al. [10]; Nessa et al. [37]; and Bhowmik et al. [7].

professionals are working with those post-stroke patients with a set of standard goals, and after achieving this goal, they send them back to the community or home to continue community-based rehabilitation services by several NGOs [10, 20, 39]. Similarly, they are continuing preventive and promotive services through NCDs corner of the primary care level to reduce the second chance of stroke attack [40]. This study concentrated only on the post-stroke out-patient rehabilitation services system in Bangladesh. According to Ahmed et al. [10], CRP is a rehabilitation center for serving post-stroke rehabilitation services in Bangladesh. It is serving hospital-based inpatient, out-patient, domiciliary, and community-based rehabilitation services. **Figure 4** shows the stroke and post-stroke care pathways along with the rehabilitation services in Bangladesh.

8. The CRP post-stroke out-patient rehabilitation services pathways

According to Runa [29], CRP is the biggest rehabilitation hospital in Bangladesh. It provides comprehensive post-stroke rehabilitation services following a Multi-Disciplinary Team (MDT) approach. The MDT team is composed of a physician, physiotherapist, occupational therapist, speech and language therapist, rehabilitation nurse, and patient's caregiver.

According to the CRP service delivery process [39], at the first contact, the patient comes to the reception (1) to collect the serial token, and after collecting the token, they have to wait in the waiting areas (2) for MDT screening (3). The MDT professionals screen the patient's condition and consequently recommend the patient for further rehabilitation services. According to the MDT recommendations, the patient goes to the laboratory (4) for the clinical test if recommended and reception

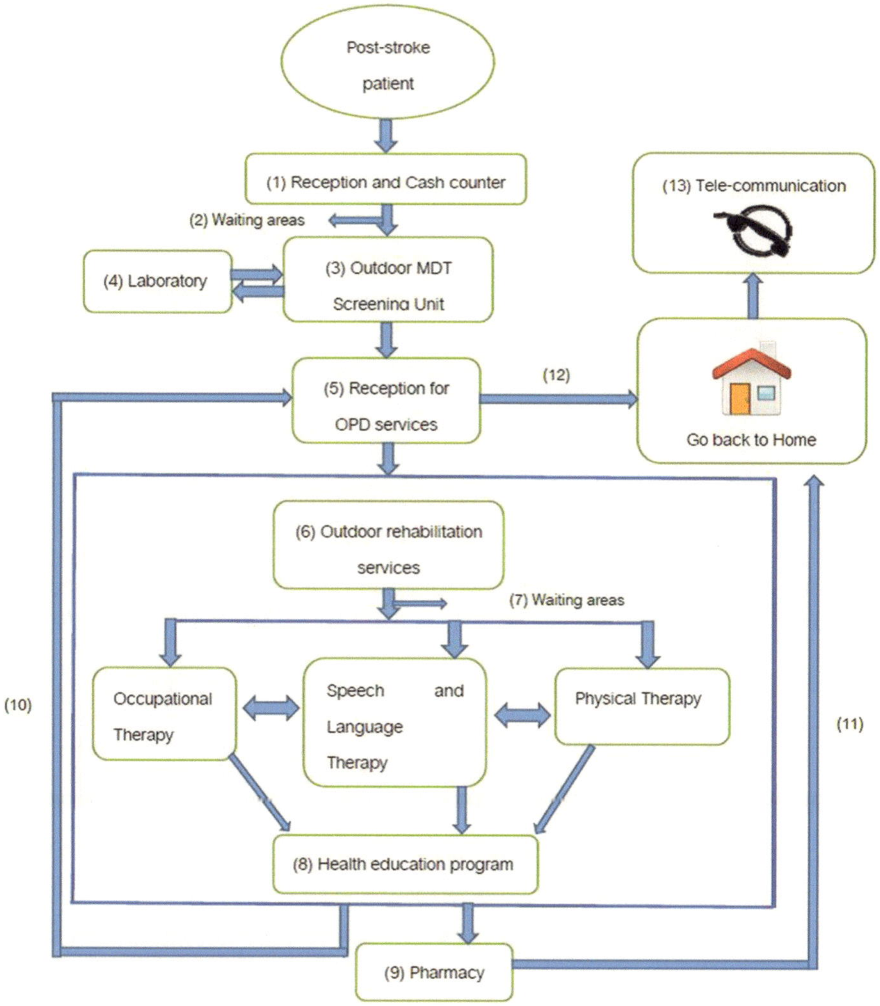

Figure 5.
Demonstrated the overall post-stroke outpatient rehabilitation services pathways in the CRP hospital. Sources and Adopted: From, CRP [39].

(5) for the appointment of outpatient rehabilitation services. There are three departments; physical therapy, occupational therapy, and speech and language therapy for post-stroke rehabilitation services. After collecting the therapists' appointment from the reception, the patient has to go to the recommended departments (6) to receive the therapy services and wait for therapy timing (7). However, the patient may have to visit several departments based on the patient's needs. The repetition of the therapy session depends on the patients' physical stability and availability of the therapy session. The three departments professional demonstrate a health education program (8) at the end of their therapy session. The main purpose of this program is to provide knowledge about stroke risk factors prevention and health promotional activities.

At the end of the session, according to the therapist's recommendation, the patient may have to go to the pharmacy (9) and the reception (10) again for further appointments. Finally, the patient goes back home (11, 12) and comes again on another day for a laboratory report and the next appointments if needed. Otherwise, the patient and the patient's caregiver can get help from CRP telemedicine services (13) and CBR services. Using this telecommunications service, they can continue their therapy services at home (**Figure 5**) [39].

9. Post-Stroke healthcare scenario of other underdeveloped and neighbor countries

9.1 India

The Republic of India is a border country of Bangladesh. India is surrounded almost entirely by sharing its' borders within west, north, and east areas. It has been following a three-tiered model of health care service delivery. These tiered models comprise of primary, secondary, and tertiary level of healthcare services. The primary healthcare centers are particularly focusing on prevention, recognition, and referral for rehabilitation. The secondary level at district hospitals has fortified with medical doctors and other general facilities. At the divisional level, all tertiary care hospitals have equipped with all specialized facilities that are provided by public and private healthcare organizations [57]. There are enormous differences in accessibility and affordability in private and public hospitals for post-stroke healthcare services. For this circumstance, it's becoming a major challenge for the patients who are seeking quality healthcare facilities for after-stroke patients.

9.2 Myanmar

The Republic of the Union of Myanmar has been sharing its border with the country of Bangladesh. Myanmar has been following pluralistic healthcare system followed by public, private, and NGO sectors. Ministry of Health (MOH) and other professional organizations have been working collaboratively for reducing communicable diseases. While communicable diseases declined, non-communicable diseases have been rising as a major concerning issue in Myanmar. The Department of Health (DOH) is mainly responsible for ensuring healthcare services through rural health centres (RHCs) and sub-rural health centres (Sub-RHCs) in the corresponding the municipality, district, and regional health centers. Preventive, promotive, and rehabilitative services have been providing for all citizens as well as for post-stroke patients to reduce premature deaths. All RHCs, Sub-RHCs are providing primary care services and at the regional level has available emergency and specialized hospital services based on the patients' need [58].

9.3 Nepal

Nepal is a state of government that has spanned a decade of political disturbance, revolution, and ferocity from the years 1996 to 2006. That particularly affects the development of healthcare sectors in Nepal. In this regard, private sectors have been following a leading role in ensuring healthcare services for the citizens of Nepal. Nepal's healthcare system is struggling to control infectious diseases and the Ministry of Health and Population (MoHP) has made a significant achievement in reducing infectious diseases. However, due to demographic changes and urbanization, the burden of national diseases has shifted from infectious to non-infectious disease patterns [59]. Wherein, 108 out of every 100,000 deaths in Nepal are occurring by cerebrovascular diseases and almost 543/100,000 persons have led a Disability-Adjusted Life Years (DALY) after their stroke [60]. Public and private sectors have been providing curative and rehabilitative services but, patients have to depend on the private sector for emergency and specialized hospital facilities. The affordability of medical treatment has considered a major role in accessing hospital facilities for all citizens. Besides, out-of-pocket payment is a very common problem in Nepal to receive in-patients hospital services.

9.4 Bhutan

The Royal Government of Bhutan provides free health care services by following the principles of primary healthcare strategy. Bhutan has improved slowly on the way to building a strong health system. However, the Ministry of Health (MoH) has faced several burdens of diseases where the prevalence of non-communicable diseases (NCDs) is aggravated. To fight against the growing trend of NCDs, Bhutan has applied a multisectoral national action plan to prevent health risks of NCDs [61].

9.5 Maldives

The Maldives is a developing country where the government is the head of the country. The Maldives has achieved a distinguished improvement in the health status of all citizens in gaining five out of eight Millennium Development Goals (MDGs) that creates a strong basement in achieving sustainable development goals (SDGs). However, considering the socioeconomic and environmental changes, the country has faced new challenges in controlling non-communicable diseases (NCDs). About 81% of total deaths are caused by NCDs in the Maldives. To address the burden of NCDs, a multisectoral national plan of action has been developed and implemented in focusing on preventive and promotional health interventions to bring changes in lifestyles and reduce health risks of NCDs. The Ministry of Health (MoH) is primarily responsible for ensuring primary health care facilities for all citizens, where, some private hospitals and NGOs provide healthcare in collaboration with the public sector. The government has spent the maximum amount of the total budget in the health sector. For instance, out-of-pocket payments for healthcare services are declining [59, 62].

10. Conclusion

The burden of NCDs as well as stroke is not an issue of a particular country. Globally, it is now a common public health concerning issue. World Health Organization has been working worldwide in dropping down the risk of NCDs.

Several countries have adopted a multisectoral collaboration approach to improve health status and work collaboratively with the participation of all individuals in different sectors. In Bangladesh, the Ministry of Health and Family Welfare in cooperation with various NGOs and private organizations has launched NCD corner at the Upazila level for providing preventive, promotional, and rehabilitative services in the community for persons who are having health risks and after-stroke disability. The scarcity of healthcare personnel is also an important barrier for providing such services. At the same time, healthcare financing and lack of infrastructure are the most important hindering factors for maintaining these kinds of services in the community. Therefore, this is the time for the ministry of health and family welfare to work with other ministries and donor agencies for the betterment of all citizens of Bangladesh.

11. The way to meet the challenges

- In order to reduce the bureaucratic problem in adopting any approach related to healthcare in society, the government has to implement a decentralization system.
- The government should increase the annual health care budget for providing low-cost or free treatment facilities. In this case, the government should work with various national and international donor agencies for financial assistance.
- Government and other legislative organizations need to work on primary care practices in both rural and urban areas by increasing the capacity of primary care workers. Similarly, it recommends considering planning environmental changes to make the infrastructure user-friendly and accessible to all.
- Local community leaders, social workers, and general people are needed to be aware of the health risk of NCDs. In this case, a multisectoral collaboration in action approach would be an effective way to work collaboratively as well as initiating telerehabilitation services, remote rehabilitation services, public education, and awareness for early rehabilitation in reducing health risks of affecting NDCs.
- Continuous quality control and monitoring systems are needed for maintaining the quality of the healthcare services as well as strengthening the healthcare service systems of Bangladesh.

Acknowledgements

Ethical approval: Not applicable. **Informed consent**: Not applicable. **Animal Studies**: Not applicable. **Funding support**: We are thankful to the Society of Speech and Language Therapists (SSLTs) in Bangladesh for their overall support to complete this article. Also, thankful to all authors those were sharing their thought and ideas to write this article.

Conflict of interest

The study authors declared that there is no conflict of interest.

Appendices and nomenclature

BRAC	Bangladesh Rehabilitation Assistance Committee
CBR	Community-Based Rehabilitation
CNS	Central Nervous System
COPD	Chronic Obstetric Pulmonary Diseases
CRP	Centre for Rehabilitation of the Paralyzed
DALY	Disability-Adjusted Life Year
DGHS	Directorate General of Health Services
DOH	Department of Health
GDP	Growth Domestic Product
HI	Handicap International
HNPSI	Health, Nutrition and Population Strategic Investment
ICH	Intracerebral Hemorrhage
ICRC	International Committee of the Red Cross
MDG	Millennium Development Goal
MDT	Multi-Disciplinary Team
MoH	Ministry of Health
MoH&FW	Ministry of Health and Family Welfare
MoHP	Ministry of Health and Population
NCD	Non-Communicable Diseases
RHC	Rural Health Centre
SAARC	South Asian Association of Regional Cooperation
SAH	Subarachnoid Hemorrhage
SDGs	Sustainable Development Goals
SEAR	South-East Asia Region
SSLTs	Society of Speech and Language Therapists
TRP	Trust for Rehabilitation of the Paralyzed
UTI	Urinary Tract Infections
WCPT	World Confederation for Physical Therapy

Author details

Mohammad Shaikhul Hasan[1,2,4*], Kanida Narattharaksha[1], Md. Sazzad Hossain[3,4] and Nahar Afrin[2,4]

1 College of Health Systems Management (CHSM), Graduate School, Naresuan University, Phitsanulok, Thailand

2 Centre for the Rehabilitation of the Paralysed (CRP), Chapain, Savar, Dhaka, Bangladesh

3 Speech and Language Therapy Department, Bangladesh Health Professions' Institute (BHPI) the Academic Institute of CRP, Chapain, Savar, Dhaka, Bangladesh

4 Members, Society of Speech and Language Therapists (SSLTs), Chapain, Savar, Dhaka, Bangladesh

*Address all correspondence to: mdshaikhulh59@email.nu.ac.th

References

[1] Hoy DG, Rao C, Hoa NP, Suhardi S, Lwin AMM. Stroke mortality variations in South-East Asia: empirical evidence from the field. International Journal of Stroke. 2013;**8**(SA100):21-27

[2] Pitthayapong S, Thiangtam W, Powwattana A, Leelacharas S, Waters CM. A community based program for family caregivers for post stroke survivors in Thailand. Asian Nursing Research. 2017;**11**(2):150-157

[3] SAARC. 2009. About South Asian Association for Regional Cooperation. Accessed: November 10, 2017, Available from: SAARC http://saarc-sec.org/about-saarc.

[4] Ministry of Health and Family Welfare. Health Bulletin 2016. Management Information System Directorate General of Health Services. Dhaka, Mohakhali: Bangladesh; 2016

[5] Bangladesh National Portal. 2018. Bangladesh Information and Services. Accessed: October 3, 2017, Available from: Bangladesh Govenment http://www.bangladesh.gov.bd/.

[6] World Bank. 2017a. Bangladesh population statistics and socio-economic status. Accessed: September 25, 2017, Avialble from: World Bank https://data.worldbank.org/country/bangladesh.

[7] Bhowmik NB, Abbas A, Saifuddin M, Islam M, Habib R, Rahman A, et al. Ischemic strokes: Observations from a hospital based stroke registry in Bangladesh. Stroke Research and Treatment. 2016;**2016**

[8] Muhammad F, Chowdhury M, Arifuzzaman M, Chowdhury AA. Public health problems in Bangladesh: Issues and challenges. South East Asia Journal of Public Health. 2017;**6**(2):11-16

[9] World Bank. 2017b. Life-expectancy at birth, total (years). Accessed: September 25, 2017, Available from: World Bank https://data.worldbank.org/indicator/SP.DYN.LE00.IN.

[10] Ahmed SM, Alam BB, Anwar I, Begum T, Huque R, Khan JA, et al. Bangladesh health system review Asia Pacific observatory on health systems and policies. Health Systems in Transition. 2015;**5**(3):1, 6, 54, 102-1, 6, 54, 118

[11] Institute for Health Metrics and Evaluation. (2016). Bangladesh. Institute for Health Metrics and Evaluation Accessed: March 15, 2017, Available From: Institute for Health Metrics and Evaluation http://www.healthdata.org/bangladesh.

[12] World Bank. 2017c. Cause of death, by non-communicable diseases (% of total). Accessed: September 25, 2017, Available from: World Bank https://data.worldbank.org/indicator/SH.DTH.NCOM.ZS?locations=BD&view

[13] Mateen F, Carone M, Alam N, Streatfield P, Black R. A population-based case–control study of 1250 stroke deaths in rural Bangladesh. European Journal of Neurology. 2012;**19**(7):999-1006

[14] Islam A. Health System in Bangladesh: Challenges and Opportunities. American Journal of Health Research. 2014;**2**(6):366. DOI: 10.11648/j.ajhr.20140206.18

[15] Sacco RL, Kasner SE, Broderick JP, Caplan LR, Connors JJ, Culebras A, et al. An updated definition of stroke for the 21st century: A statement for healthcare professionals from the American Heart Association/

American Stroke Association. Stroke. 2013;**44**(7):2064-2089. DOI: 10.1161/STR.0b013e318296aeca

[16] Kobylańska M, Wójcik BM, Szczepaniak R, Śliwiński Z. The rehabilitation of patients after the cerebral stroke including socio-demographic factors. Fizjoterapia Polska. 2016;**16**(4):82-97

[17] American Heart Association. American Heart Association Annual Statistical Update Report on Heart and Stroke Health. American Heart Association; 2017 Accessed: April 12, 2017, American Heart Association http://newsroom.heart.org/news/new-statistical-update-looks-at-worldwide-heart-stroke-health

[18] Australian Institute of Health and Welfare. (2016). Heart, stroke, and vascular diseases. Australian Institute of Health and Welfare. Accessed: April 5, 2017, Available from: Australian Government https://www.aihw.gov.au/reports-statistics/health-conditions-disability-deaths/heart-stroke-vascular-diseases/overview.

[19] Van Exel N, Koopmanschap M, Scholte op Reimer, W., Niessen, L. W., & Huijsman, R. Cost-effectiveness of integrated stroke services. QJM. 2005;**98**(6):415-425

[20] Islam MN, Moniruzzaman M, Khalil MI, Basri R, Alam MK, Loo KW, et al. Burden of stroke in Bangladesh. International Journal of Stroke. 2013;**8**(3):211-213. DOI: 10.1111/j.1747-4949.2012.00885.x

[21] Global Health Statistics. 2017. Stroke in Bangladesh. Statistics on Overall Impact and Specific Effect on Demographic Groups. Accessed: October 30, 2017, Available from: Health Grove http://global-disease-burden.healthgrove.com/l/42217/Stroke-in-Bangladesh.

[22] Mohammad Q. Management of stroke-Bangladesh perspective. Bangladesh Medical Journal. 2014;**42**(1):34-37

[23] Centre for Injury Prevention Health Development and Research Bangladesh (CIPRB). 2014. Prevalence of stroke in the rural community of Bangladesh. Accessed: March 3, 2017, Available from: CIPRB evidance for quality life http://www.ciprb.org/prevalence-of-stroke-in-the-rural-community-of-bangladesh/.

[24] Mamin FA, Islam MS, Rumana FS, Faruqui F. Profile of stroke patients treated at a rehabilitation centre in Bangladesh. BMC Research Notes. 2017;**10**(1):520. DOI: 10.1186/s13104-017-2844-x

[25] American Stroke Association. 2012. Effects of Stroke. Accessed: March 5, 2017, American Stroke Association Available from: https://www.strokeassociation.org/STROKEORG/AboutStroke/EffectsofStroke/Effects-of-Stroke_UCM_308534_SubHomePage.jsp.

[26] Wolfe CD. The impact of stroke. British Medical Bulletin. 2000;**56**(2):275-286

[27] National Stroke Association. 2017. Rehabilitation Therapy After Stroke. Accessed: March 3, 2017, Available from: National Stroke Association www.stroke.org.com.

[28] Gordon NF, Gulanick M, Costa F, Fletcher G, Franklin BA, Roth EJ, et al. Physical activity and exercise recommendations for stroke survivors: An American Heart Association scientific statement from the Council on Clinical Cardiology, Subcommittee on Exercise, Cardiac Rehabilitation, and Prevention; the Council on Cardiovascular Nursing; the Council on Nutrition, Physical Activity, and Metabolism; and the Stroke Council. Stroke. 2004;**35**(5):1230-1240

[29] Runa SA. The common secondary complications among the stroke patients at crp. Dhaka, Bangladesh: Bangladesh Health Professions Institute, Faculty of Medicine, the University of Dhaka, Bangladesh; 2015

[30] Anhang Price R, Elliott MN, Zaslavsky AM, Hays RD, Lehrman WG, Rybowski L, et al. Examining the role of patient experience surveys in measuring health care quality. Medical Care Research and Review. 2014;**71**(5):522-554. DOI: 10.1177/1077558714541480

[31] Akachi Y, Tarp F, Kelley E, Addison T, Kruk ME. Measuring quality-of-care in the context of sustainable development goal 3: a call for papers. Bulletin of the World Health Organization. 2016;**94**(3):160

[32] Burazeri G, Kragelj LZ. Health: Systems-lifestyle-policies. In: A Handbook for Teachers, Researchers and Health Professionals. 2nd ed. Detmold, Germany: Jacobs Verlag Publishers; 2013. pp. 393-416

[33] WHO. 2000. The World Health Report 2000- Health systems: improving performance. Accessed: June 19, 2017, Available from: WHO http://www.who.int/whr/2000/en/.

[34] Ministry of Law. The Constitution of The People's Republic of Bangladesh. Bangladesh: Ministry of Law, Justice and Parliamentary Affairs; 2010

[35] Rahman DMS. 2016. Healthcare Delivery Systems in Bangladesh. Accessed: September 20, 2017, Available from: The Health & Medicine https://www.slideshare.net/rahmanshuvo10/health-care-delivery-system-in-bangladesh-1234.

[36] Ahmad A. Provision of Primary Healthcare Services in Urban areas of Bangladesh–the Case of Urban Primary Health Care Project. Department of Economics: Lund University, Lund; 2007

[37] Nessa J, Khaleque MA, Begum S, Ahmed AH, Islam S, Afsan M. Rehabilitation of stroke patients-effects of early intervention of physical therapy on functional outcome. Bangladesh Journal of Anatomy. 2009;**7**(1):62-67

[38] Roy T. 2015. Centre for the Rehabilitation of the Paralysed [Press release]. Available from: http://en.banglapedia.org/index.php?title=Centre_for_the_Rehabilitation_of_the_Paralysed.

[39] CRP. 2017. CRP at a Glance. Accessed: November 20, 2017, Available from: CRP http://www.crp-bangladesh.org.

[40] Biswas T, Pervin S, Tanim MIA, Niessen L, Islam A. Bangladesh policy on prevention and control of non-communicable diseases: a policy analysis. BMC Public Health. 2017;**17**(1):582. DOI: 10.1186/s12889-017-4494-2

[41] Ministry of Health and Family Welfare. Health Bulletin 2015. Management Information System Directorate General of Health Services, Bangladesh: Dhaka, Mohakhali; 2015

[42] World Confederation for Physical Therapy (WCPT). 2017. Bangladesh: A profile of the profession. Accessed: November 16, 2017, Available from: WCPT http://www.wcpt.org/node/26376/cds.

[43] BHPI. Bangladesh Health Professions Institute (BHPI), An Academic Institute of CRP. 2017. Available from: https://wwwbhpiedubd/

[44] SSLTs. Society of Speech and Language Therapists (SSLTs). Dhaka, Bangladesh. Annual Report 2016-2017. 2017;2

[45] Accounts BNH. Tracking Urban Health Expenditures—Preliminary Results from Secondary Analysis of Bangladesh National Health Accounts.

USAID, Bangladesh: Health Finance & Governance; 2015

[46] Ministry of Health and Family Welfare. Strategic Plan for Surveillance and Prevention of Non-Communicable Diseases in Bangladesh 2007-2010. Directorate General of Health Services: WHO Country Office of Bangladesh; 2007

[47] Axelsson C. Mapping Report of Physical Rehabilitation Services in Afghanistan, Bangladesh, Odisha (India) and Sri Lanka. Handicap International; 2014

[48] Handicap International (HI). 2017. Community-Based Rehabilitation. Bangladesh Branch. Accessed: November 17, 2017, Available from: HI website.

[49] International Committee of the Red Cross (ICRC). 2014. Physical Rehabilitation. ICRC Bangladesh Delegation. Accessed: November 17, 2017, Available from: ICRC https://www.icrc.org/eng/assets/files/publications/icrc-002-0126t.pdf.

[50] Gresham GE, Alexander D, Bishop DS, Giuliani C, Goldberg G, Holland A, et al. Rehabilitation. Stroke. 1997;**28**(7):1522-1526

[51] Licitra L, Keilholz U, Tahara M, Lin JC, Chomette P, Ceruse P, et al. Evaluation of the benefit and use of multidisciplinary teams in the treatment of head and neck cancer. Oral Oncology. 2016;**59**:73-79. DOI: 10.1016/j.oraloncology.2016.06.002

[52] Rønning OM, Guldvog B. Outcome of subacute stroke rehabilitation: A randomized controlled trial. Stroke. 1998;**29**(4):779-784

[53] Directorate General of Health Services. Stroke Management Guideline. Dhaka: Directorate General of Health Services; 2008

[54] Mcmahon M. 2017. What is the difference between acute and sub-acute rehabilitation. Accessed: June 3, 2017, from wise week. Available from: http://www.wisegeek.org/what-is-the-difference-between-acute-and-subacute-rehabilitation.htm.

[55] National Institutes of Health. 2014. Post-Stroke Rehabilitation. Accessed: March 23, 2017, Available from: National Institutes of Health https://stroke.nih.gov/materials/rehabilitation.htm.

[56] Brodsky J, Habib J, Hirschfeld MJ, World Health Organization & WHO Collaborating Centre for Health and Long-Term Care Policy and Research. In: Brodsky J, Habib J, Hirschfeld M, editors. Long-Term Care in Developing Countries: Ten Case Studies. China: World Health Organization; 2003. https://apps.who.int/iris/handle/10665/42769

[57] Pandian JD, Sudhan P. Stroke epidemiology and stroke care services in India. Journal of Stroke. 2013;**15**:128-134. DOI: 10.5853/jos.2013.15.3.128

[58] World Health Organization. The Republic of the Union of Myanmar health system review. Manila: WHO Regional Office for the Western Pacific; 2014

[59] World Health Organization. 2018a. WHO country cooperation strategy 2018-2022: Nepal.

[60] Shakya D, Shrestha R, Dhungana K, Kafle R, Bhatta S. Ischemic stroke: Observations and analysis of stroke patients admitted in a tertiary hospital of Kathmandu. Journal of Kathmandu

Medical College. 2019;**8**(2):66-71. DOI: 10.3126/jkmc.v8i2.28166

[61] World Health Organization. 2019. WHO country cooperation strategy 2020-2024: towards transition: Bhutan.

[62] World Health Organization. 2018b. Maldives-WHO: country cooperation strategy 2018-2022.

Chapter 3

Post-Stroke Balance Impairments Assessment: Clinical Scales and Current Technologies

Paulina Ortega-Bastidas, Britam Gómez, Karen Barriga, Francisco Saavedra and Pablo Aqueveque

Abstract

This chapter aims to address the different impairments in the balance after stroke, beginning with an introduction on the main dysfunctions that can be observed, specifically in different transfers as sit-to-stand and gait. Also, a review of the main test and assessment scales most used in the clinical settings in this population. Finally, the application of new technologies and the technological advances used in clinical settings for human analysis focusing on balance are addressed. For example, the types of technologies used, their applications, and the combination with the existing clinical assessment tools. As a closure, we explain the importance of early detection and treatment of balance impairments in the post-stroke population to prevent falls.

Keywords: balance, impairments, stroke, assessment, technology

1. Introduction

All functional activities performed by human beings require adequate postural control to carry them out successfully and efficiently. Postural control is the ability to maintain balance against gravitational forces by maintaining or returning the body mass center on its base support [1, 2]. This emerges from the interaction between subjects, tasks, and environment [2, 3]. Any task requires adequate postural control, but each task also requires an orientation and a stability component [2].

In clinical practices, there is no consensus about only conceptual definitions related to equilibrium, balance, or postural control, and their elements like posture, orientation, and stability. Therefore, it is interesting to at least define basic biomechanical concepts to better understand postural control and further definitions addressed in this chapter.

From a biomechanical point of view, posture refers to the alignment and orientation of the body with respect to its environment [3]. Postural orientation is the ability to maintain an adequate relation between body segments and environment due to performing a task, and postural stability is the ability to control the center of mass within the base support [2, 3].

IntechOpen

Nowadays, postural control is no longer considered as only one system or reflex set for upright position and balance, it is considered a complex motor skill due to the interaction of multiple sensorimotor processes [4]. The two main goals of postural control are keeping postural orientation and postural equilibrium [2–4].

The human body in order to achieve stability and orientation requires a complex interaction between musculoskeletal components, neuromuscular synergies, individual sensory systems, sensory strategies, anticipatory and adaptive mechanisms, and internal representations [2]. The central nervous system (CNS) must organize the information coming from the different sensory receptors to determine the position of the body in space [2]. The sensory information coming from the different sensory systems (visual, somatosensory, and vestibular) allows to detect the position of the body and the movement in space in relation to the force of gravity and the environment [2, 3, 5]. Each sense provides specific information about the position and movement of the body, that is, each sense provides different references for postural control [2]. In the higher levels, the CNS sensory information is transformed into significative information, known as perception, and then it is selected the best sensorimotor strategies to achieve the goal of a specific task, to control external perturbance, and to adapt movement to the environmental requirements [2].

Also, postural orientation involves active control of alignment and tone of the body related to gravity, base support, visual information, and internal references [2, 3]. Spatial orientation requires the interpretation and integrated information of the visual, vestibular, and somatosensory systems. On the other hand, postural equilibrium involves the coordination of sensorimotor strategies to control the center of mass during internal and external disturbances [3, 4]. For a better explanation of the different sensory systems and sensory strategies to maintain postural control, see the diagram in **Figure 1**.

There are multiple causes and factors that could lead to dysfunctions in postural control and balance systems. In neurological populations, is commonly observed that

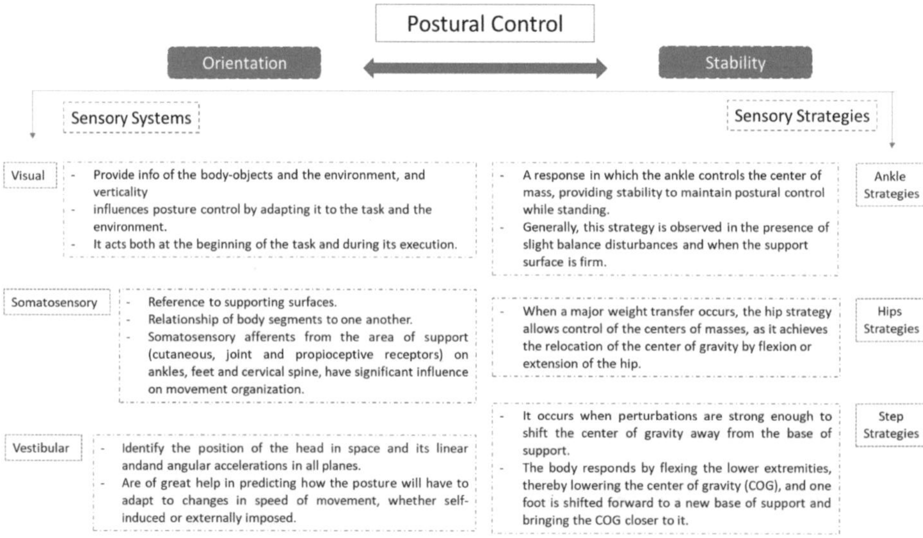

Figure 1.
Postural control by sensory systems and strategies. Summary information collected from Shumway-Cook and Woollacott [2], Cano de La Cuerda [3], Cano de la Cuerda and Callado Vasquez [5].

this deficit affects the ability to stand and walk, increasing the risk of falling and injury [2].

Within neurological populations, we can find stroke patients. Stroke is a common disease [6] that generates great morbidity, mortality, and different degrees of disability, causing a great economic impact on families and society [1].

A stroke can lead to a wide range of impairments that predispose the subjects to falls. One of the principal impairments observed in this population is balance dysfunction [7, 8]. It has been reported that 83% of stroke patients present balance impairments, which lead to gait problems, such as low gait speed and alterations in different gait phases increasing the risk of falling [1]. The incidence of falls in this population within the first six months after a stroke is about 37 and 73%, and the rate of falls in chronic stroke patients is double than healthy subjects [8].

Falls and fear of falling contribute to a sedentary lifestyle with increased limitations in activities of daily living (ADL) and decreased quality of life. In addition, falls increase hospitalization time and generate a large emotional and economic impact for patients, families, and society [1, 9, 10].

The present chapter pretends to expose the principal deficiencies related to balance impairments, observed during the sit-to-stand transfer and gait after a stroke. Also, the main scales and tests for the assessments of balance used in clinical settings, as well as the technologies and new trends that allow for objective analysis of balance dysfunction in this population are reviewed.

2. Principals balance impairments after stroke

As said before, postural control alterations contribute to a loss of stability with a high impact on the quality of life in neurological populations [1, 2]. Balance and postural control impairments cause a series of alterations and dysfunctions during daily life activities, mainly during sit-to-stand transfer and gait [11, 12].

In this section, the main alterations on the sit-to-stand transfer as well as in gait related to balance impairments in post-stroke populations are reviewed.

2.1 Impairments in sit-to-stand transfer after stroke

Sit-to-stand (STS) transfer is considered a fundamental prerequisite to achieve successfully daily life activities [11–13]. Also, it is considered a strong predictor factor of independence and is the main rehabilitation goal because it promotes independent locomotion, as well as upper limb and hand recovery [13]. In post-stroke populations, this transfer is commonly affected, and it is not easy to regain the ability to stand up from a chair safely [11].

The STS transfer has been widely analyzed [11, 14, 15], and has been described as the movement of the body mass center towards the vertical from a sitting position to an upright position without losing balance [11]. This transfer is a transition to the upright position, and it requires a movement of the mass center from a more stable position into a less one with both lower limbs extended [11, 15]. In order to simplify its analysis, the STS transfer has been divided into phases, depending on kinematics variables, ground action forces, and the movement of the mass center [11].

One of these classifications includes four phases for the analysis, considering trunk movement, seat-off, the achievement of an upright position, and the vertical stabilization at the end of the transfer [11]. Another classification considers two principal phases [11, 15], which basically includes three events, onset of STS, seat-off, and end of STS [15].

Associated with this transfer, there have been described different movement determinants in healthy subjects, such as angular displacements of lower limbs and trunk, as well as muscle activation pattern and weight-bearing distribution [16].

Indeed, there are differences in the performance of sit-to-stand transfer between healthy and post-stroke subjects [11, 13–15].

Normally, people with hemiparesis show a loss of coordinated movement between the trunk and knees. Therefore, it can be observed a completed knee extension at the end of the STS despite the hip it is still extending. Also, they show an increased center of pressure and move the trunks in a mediolateral direction towards the non-paretic side, as well as a decreased anterior pelvic tilt [11, 15, 16]. When observed lower limbs, it can be identified less muscle activity in the paretic limb, specifically of tibialis anterior, quadriceps, and soleus, showing problems in the correct activation muscle timing to achieve STS [11, 15].

To avoid the risk of falling, people with stroke adopt compensatory strategies, such as exaggeration of the anterior projection of the center of mass before standing up. This population also shows a decrease in knee moment on the paretic side and an increase in weight distribution asymmetry [11, 15, 16]. It has been suggested a correlation between asymmetry in weight-bearing with functional abilities in stroke. It states that those who carry less weight on their paretic limb obtain poor mobility scores in the functional independence scales. These same results have been demonstrated by Cheng et al. who consider the asymmetric distribution of weight-bearing during STS as a mediator of falls [11, 16].

All of these compensatory strategies are carried out to achieve the sit-to-stand transfer successfully and safely, but this population takes more time in the execution of this task, increasing the risk of falling. Because of the big amount of compensatory strategies used by the stroke population, this transfer is considered an indicator of the risk of falling [11, 16].

2.2 Principal gait impairments after stroke

Similar to STS, independent walking or ambulation is also considered a prerequisite for the performance of activities of daily living [14]. Gait requires an adequate speed to be considered community ambulation, between 1.1 and 1.5 m/s [14]. Also, locomotion is a motor skill, in which control systems in every step must bear weight, give anterior and lateral stability, and keep the center of mass forward, as well as an antigravitatory postural control to provide support and balance to prevent falls [10, 11, 14].

Gait dysfunction represents a major problem in the stroke population and causes difficulties in daily life activities [12, 17]. Approximately 80% of stroke patients experience gait problems in the first 3 months after symptom onset. It has been reported that 18% of subjects are unable to walk, while 11% walk with assistance and the remaining 50% walk independently [12]. It is important to note that only 7% of users who walk independently achieve community walking, which means that they manage to walk 500 meters continuously at an adequate walking speed that allows them to cross the street safely [16].

On the other hand, 70% of stroke patients with community walking suffer falls in the first year, most of these falls are the result of loss in balance. Therefore, there is a high risk of falls in those subjects with stroke who walk independently [12].

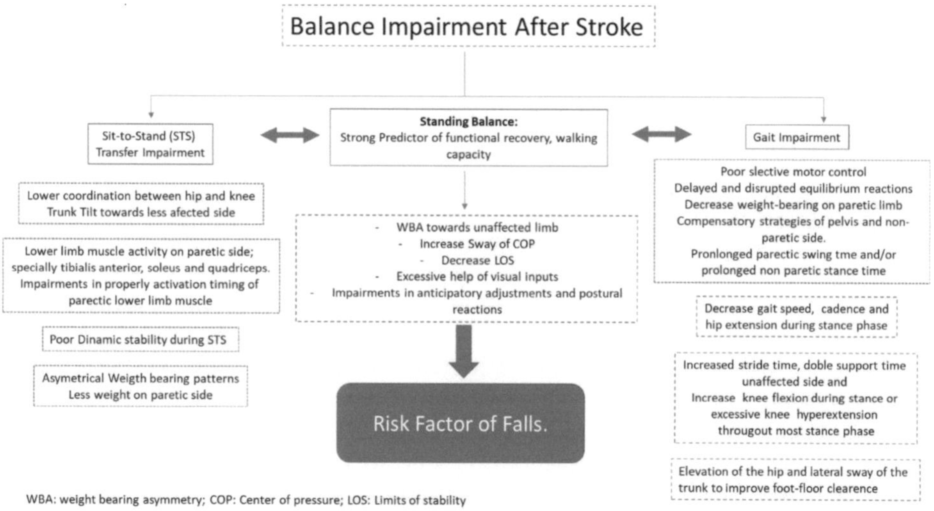

Figure 2.
Balance and gait impairments after stroke. Summary information collected from Boukadida et al. [11], Perry [17], Dickstein [18], Wang et al. [19] Hugues et al. [22], Van Duijnhoven [23], Silva et al. [24], Brière et al. [25], Balandan [26].

Post-stroke gait disturbances and their treatment have been extensively researched [12, 18–20]. Mainly, we could find impairments associated with alterations in spatial-temporal characteristics and biomechanical alterations [12, 19].

Some of the characteristics of hemiparetic gait related to spatiotemporal variables include decreased cadence, prolonged swing duration on the paretic side, prolonged duration on the nonparetic side, and asymmetry in stride length [19]. As well as the increase of the double support phase and the decrease in gait speed [16, 19].

These characteristics contribute to an unsteady gait pattern, leading to restricted walking within the home and an increased risk of falls [21].

In general, due to a stroke, we can observe different impairments that may occur in the paretic lower extremity, such as abnormal recruitment of motor units, muscle weakness, abnormal activation of muscle synergies, spasticity, proprioceptive impairment, restriction in range of motion, which could enhance a poor gait pattern along with balance disturbances and increased risk of falls [13, 18, 22].

Figure 2 shows the main features in balance impairments related to sit-to-stand, standing balance, and gait after stroke. It is important to highlight that there are more features related to each transfer, but we aim to clarify the most common one in this population.

3. Tests and scales for static and dynamic equilibrium assessment

Nowadays, it has become relevant to observe the quality of the movement patterns to discriminate between actual recovery and compensatory movement patterns in stroke rehabilitation [10]. Balance impairments are common in this population and they are determinants factor that influences independence and quality of life; therefore, balance became an important goal to be included in rehabilitation programs [21]. For this purpose, the use of accurate, reliable, and valid assessment tools to measure outcomes in stroke populations related to research and clinical practice is recommended [7].

Normally, rehabilitation professionals perform the evaluation by means of observation and the application of scales and instruments, which provide a certain level of objectivity [27]. Generally, the different methodology used for assessing balance can be divided into observational (e.g., the Romberg test), scales and tests, and testing instrumental equipment (e.g., posturography) [28].

The Berg balance scale (BBS) is a widely used tool in clinical settings and is considered the gold standard for assessing functional balance and fall risk in adults [2, 3, 21, 29]. It has been used extensively to measure outcomes in research involving older adults with a variety of conditions, for example, balance impairments, stroke, Parkinson's disease, vestibular disorders, and in a variety of health care settings [30–32]. It contains 14 items related to the static and dynamic tasks of daily living [3]. The tasks on this scale progress in difficulty from sitting to bipedal, to bipedal with a narrow support base, to tandem gait and one leg support. The score is calculated on a 5-point ordinal scale for each item, where 0 refers to the inability to complete the test and 4 refers to being able to complete the test independently [3, 29]. The maximum score is 56 points that indicates adequate postural balance and no risk of falls, and a score equal to or less than 45 points indicates a risk of falls [3]. Specifically, values between 56 and 41 points indicate a low risk of falling, between 40 and 21 points a medium risk of falling, and between 20 and 0 points a high risk of falling. Its application lasts between 10 and 20 minutes [29–32]. Another widely used test is the Timed up and Go (TU & Go) test, which measures dynamic balance and functional mobility in adults, as well as in the neurological population [33–35]. The TU & Go is a simple test that can be applied anywhere and consists of the subject standing up from a chair, walking three meters, turning around, walking back to the chair, and sitting down on the chair again. The controlled variable is the total time in seconds the subject takes to perform the test, which is then correlated with the risk of falling [34–36]. Score assumed to be normal if the time is $\leq$10 seconds, mild risk of falling between 11 and 20 seconds, and high risk >20 seconds [37]. This test has demonstrated excellent inter- and intra-rater reliability with values greater than 0.95, with adequate predictive value for falls in older adults and stroke patients [38, 39]. Some advantages of the TU & Go test are its simplicity and short duration of application. Additionally, it requires little equipment and allows subjects with functional impairment to perform the test [3]. However, one limitation is that although it provides information on the risk of falls, it is not able to determine the risk objectively in subjects with greater difficulties. Barry et al. mention that a limitation in the predictive value of the test could be explained by the fact that it is a single test that evaluates balance and equilibrium in a general way. Therefore, it could be improved by being combined with technological tools for motion analysis [40].

Commonly, in clinical practice, this test is combined with the application of other clinical tests such as the 10-meter walk test, and its results are compared with those obtained in the Berg balance scale [30]. These tests as a whole make it possible to assess the risk of falls, walking speed, and balance of the different patients, making it possible to objectively assess their functional level and to determine the relevant intervention strategies.

Gait speed has been shown to be a predictor for different clinical outcomes, such as response to rehabilitation, level of dependency, frailty, disability, falls, institutionalization, cognitive loss, hospitalization, cardiovascular events, and mortality. Its decrease has been associated with a lower quality of life, social participation, and the presence of depressive symptoms [41]. Middleton et al. define it as the sixth vital sign due to its broad predictive capacity. The 10-meter walk test has proven to be a robust, validated, reliable, and sensitive tool that can be applied in both clinical and research contexts, and in a wide range of pathologies, such as the elderly, chronic stroke, incomplete spinal cord injury, multiple sclerosis, Parkinson's disease, among others [18, 38, 41, 42].

This test measures walking speed in meters per second (m/s) when walking a short distance of 10 meters. Then, the value obtained will be categorized into the four categories proposed by Perry et. Al, which are intra-domicile gait with speeds between 0 to 0.4 ms; dependent community gait with speeds from 0.4 to 0.8 m/s; community gait 0.8 to 1.2 m/s; and safe gait for crossing the street greater than 1.2 m/s [43].

On the other hand, there is the Functional Reach Scale. This scale was developed to assess the maximum limits of standing stability. Subjects are held in a standing position with feet shoulder-width apart and with one arm (hand grasped) elevated to 90 degrees of flexion. Without moving the feet, the patient is asked to reach as far as possible without losing balance. The distance reached is measured and compared with standardized references by age group as defined by Duncan et al. The functional reach test has satisfactory inter-rater reliability and has been reported as a predictor of falls in older adults [2, 3].

Table 1 summarizes some specific characteristics of the tests and scales listed before.

Test/scale	Aim	Area	Assessment	Description	Cost	Duration
Berg balance scale [3, 44]	Static balance and risk of falling.	Balance, functional mobility.	Performance measurement (score).	Scale that considers 14 items that include static and dynamic activities of varying difficulty. Each activity is evaluated from 0 to 4 points, determined by the patient's ability to perform the activity in question. Maximum score 56.	Free (Paper and pencil)	10 to 20 min.
Timed up and go [37, 44]	Risk of falling.	Balance, functional mobility, vestibular assessment.	Observer.	Subject begins seated with his back against the back of a chair. At the beginning of the test, the patient gets up from the chair and walks 3 meters, and then turns and returns to the starting point and sits down. The time taken to complete the circuit is recorded.	Free (paper and pencil)	≤3 min.
10-M walk test [43, 44]	Independence level.	Mobility, gait, vestibular assessment.	Performance measurement (gait speed).	Subject walks a predetermined distance (depending on the variation applied), in which time is measured. The distance walked in meters is divided by the measured time.	Free (paper and pencil)	≤ 5 min.

Test/scale	Aim	Area	Assessment	Description	Cost	Duration
Tinetti [44]	Balance perception and stability during daily life activities.	Daily life activities, Balance, Functional Mobility, Gait, and Vestibular Assessment.	Patients perception.	10-item questionnaire designed to assess patient confidence in performing 10 activities of daily living without risk of falling as an indicator of how fear of falling impacts physical performance. The higher the score (100 max) the lower the patient's confidence.	Free (paper and pencil)	10 to 15 min.
BESTest [44–46]	Postural stability and balance.	Balance, functional mobility, vestibular assessment.	Performance measurement (score).	Orients and identifies the six balance control systems in order to design better approaches to balance rehabilitation from 35 items in six sections, evaluated from 0 to 108 points.	Free (paper and pencil)	10 to 20 min.
Activities of Balance confidence (ABC) scale [44]	Self-reporting of the balance confidence measure.	Balance, functional mobility.	Patients perception.	Subjective measure of confidence to perform various ambulatory activities without falling or experiencing feelings of instability out of 16 activities scored from 0 (no confidence) to 100 (confidence).	Free (paper and pencil)	5 to 10 min.

Table 1.
Test and scale for the assessment of balance in stroke populations.

One of the most recent scales to measure balance is the Balance Evaluation Systems Test (BESTest), which is a balance assessment scale that allows identifying specific problems in postural control, such as biomechanical alterations, stability limits, postural response, anticipatory postural adjustments, sensory orientation, dynamic balance during gait, and cognitive effects. Although it is a new multitask scale, it includes 36 items to be evaluated with an estimated application time of 30 to 35 minutes [2, 3, 45, 46]. Its short version, the Mini-Balance Evaluation Systems Test (Mini-BESTest), was created in 2010, which contemplates 14 items and takes a total of 10 minutes to complete the assessment, with good inter- and intra-rater reliability in a sample of people with mixed conditions. The mini-BESTest has been shown to be a reliable and validated tool for assessing balance in chronic stroke patients [47].

As can be seen in this section, there is a wide range of scales and clinical tests that allow not only to assess balance but also to observe how the different components behave during the performance of different tasks. Some of them are not only validated in populations with stroke. Therefore, the reader is suggested to review the specific psychometric properties of each of them and their validation in other neurological populations before using it.

4. Balance impairment treatments after stroke

There are different therapeutic interventions to improve balance after stroke. According to Stein et al. [21] these interventions could be categorized into five main areas, exercise programs, biofeedback training, sensory training, cognitive training, and external devices.

Each of these areas will address different aspects of the multiple problems that can be found associated with balance impairments [21, 22]. Exercise programs are varied in form, maybe individual or group-based, and include a variety of impairment-oriented elements. Some may include functional activities such as sit-to-stand and balance tasks due to daily life activities, for example, reaching and standing on unstable surfaces [21].

Also, there are different intervention models such as constraint-induced therapy, task-oriented approach, as well as neurophysiological intervention approach such as the Bobath concept, proprioceptive neuromuscular facilitation, and other neurodevelopment models, which have been traditionally used in the treatment of post-stroke patients [5].

The incorporation of visual and sensory training has been shown to be effective in the treatment of balance, as well as the promotion of weight-bearing in seated and upright positions [21–23, 48]. On the other hand, the incorporation of therapeutic strategies that involve trunk work in the recovery of dynamic balance during sitting, sit-to-stand, and gait is relevant [49].

Since, trunk function has been associated with gait and balance ability in stroke patients and has been shown to be a useful predictor of recovery of gait, balance, and activities of daily living [49].

Recently, a meta-analysis by Hugues et al. concluded that physical therapy has various benefits on postural balance and stability after stroke. It suggests that functional task training, associated with musculoskeletal and/or cardiopulmonary interventions, as well as sensory interventions, appear to be effective in improving balance and postural stability. However, the authors ask for caution with this result, due to "the weak methodological quality of studies," among other methodological elements [21, 42].

Even though there are several therapeutic approaches and categories of physical therapy, we believe it is important to highlight that each exercise program should be individualized according to the individual's own capabilities and should be supervised by a therapist.

5. Technological tools and systems for the evaluation and treatment in post-stroke patients

5.1 Technological tools for monitoring and for the diagnostic support of post-stroke patients

At a commercial level, a large number of technological systems allow to evaluate different aspects of gait, balance, and strength beyond the typical clinical methodologies, as seen in the previous section.

From the perspective of systems that are capable of evaluating movement and even mobility variables for clinical use, there are camera-based motion analysis laboratories whose measurement is carried out using software for motion analysis (**Figure 3**).

On the other hand, in the last 30 years, there has been an increase in the use of inertial sensors for motion analysis, whose reduction in size and consumption, in addition to the improvement in algorithms for motion tracking, have allowed them to be positioned as an attractive alternative for the study of movement objectively and quantitatively (**Figure 4**).

Some other commercial alternatives are illustrated in **Table 2**.

Another type of element is highly used in the clinical field for the evaluation of gait and static and dynamic balance correspond to systems that measure plantar pressures for the estimation of mobility variables. Technological alternatives range from highly accurate mats for gait and balance evaluation, to systems that embed pressure sensors within insoles to evaluate uncontrolled environments (**Figure 5**).

Some other examples are illustrated in **Table 3**.

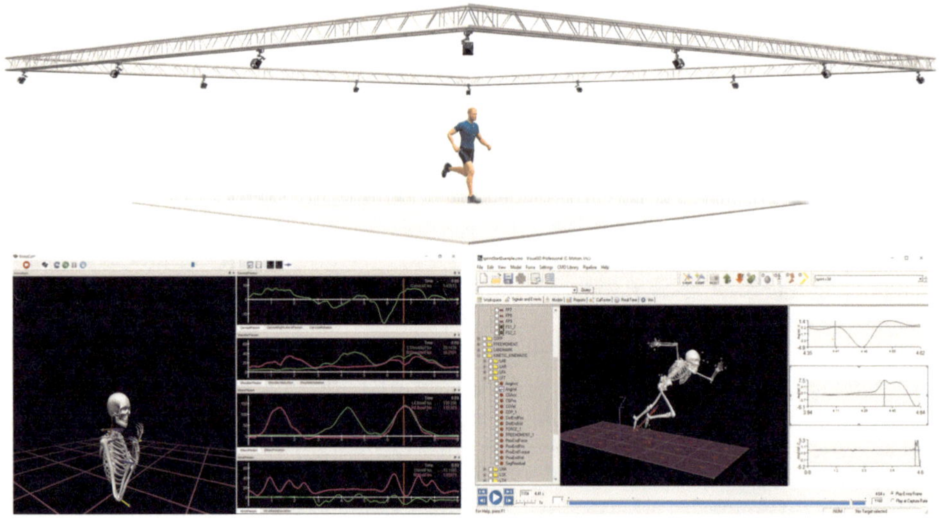

Figure 3.
Optitrack system for human motion analysis using a camera-based system. Image obtained from Optitrack official website [50].

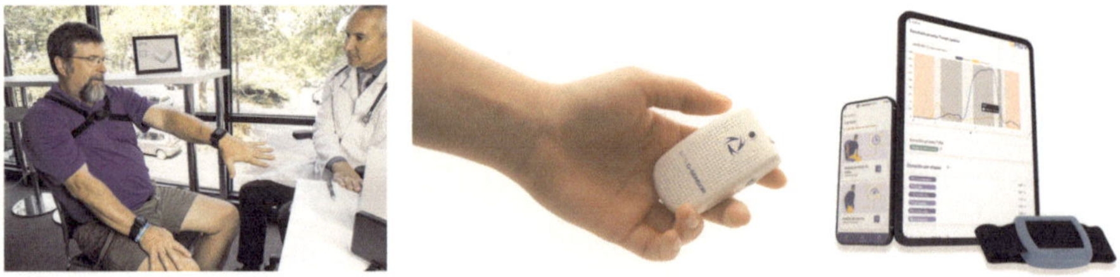

Figure 4.
Inertial-based systems for a clinical movement analysis perspective. From left to right: APDM mobility lab, G-walk, and QMUV. Images obtained from the official website of G-walk [51], APDM [52], and QMUV [63].

System	Technology	Description	Area
Vicon [54]	Optic	Leading optical system in motion analysis used in both clinical and entertainment applications. It incorporates the ability to track reflective passive markers and, together with its tracking platform, it is possible to capture the movement made by people. Using its proprietary software, such as NEXUS, clinical biomechanical and sports motion analysis can be performed. It also offers the possibility of performing biomechanical analysis by incorporating other analysis software, such as Biomechanics of Bodies.	Clinical, sports, entertainment, academic
Optitrack [50]	Optic	Optical system that incorporates a flexible system to perform biomechanical motion analysis, providing the possibility of natively incorporating other commonly used tools for motion analysis such as electromyography modules, force platforms, and analog sensors. Incorporates the ability to track passive reflective and active markers. It allows the use of other analysis software commonly used in the academic research area such as in Visual3D, The MotionMonitor, MATLAB, and Biomechanics of Bodies.	Clinical, sports, entertainment, academic
MTw Awinda – X-SENS [55]	Inertial	System with inertial technology that incorporates the possibility of evaluating variables of acceleration, speed, and ranges of movement of some segments or the whole body including hands and phalanges. It offers the possibility of performing biomechanical analysis by incorporating other analysis software such as Biomechanics of Bodies.	Clinical, sports, entertainment, academic
Perception Neuron – NOITOM [56]	Inertial	System with inertial technology that incorporates the possibility of evaluating variables of acceleration, speed, and ranges of movement of some segments or the whole body including hands and phalanges. It offers the possibility of performing biomechanical analysis by incorporating other analysis software such as Biomechanics of Bodies.	Entertainment, academic
Ultium Motion – Noraxon [57]	Inertial	System with inertial technology that incorporates the possibility of evaluating variables of acceleration, speed, and ranges of movement of some segments or the whole body with a maximum of 16 sensors.	Clinical, sports, entertainment
G-WALK [51]	Inertial	Sensorization of several clinical tests with a single inertial sensor to assess gait, balance, ranges of motion, and risk of falls. In addition to the incorporation of evaluation of aspects of sports performance such as jumping power and aerobic resistance.	Clinical, sports, academic
MobilityLab – APDM [52]	Inertial	Matrix of six inertial sensors that measure different aspects of gait and risk of falls.	Clinical, academic
QMUV [53]	Inertial	Sensorization of several clinical tests with a single inertial sensor to assess gait, balance, ranges of motion, and risk of falls.	Clinical, academic

Table 2.
Commercial technological alternatives used to evaluate motor impairment conditions in post-stroke patients.

System	Description	Area
Xsensor [58]	Insoles with plantar pressure points to measure gait variables in sports and clinical applications.	Clinical, sports
Moticon [60]	Insole for gait analysis in rehabilitation and sports training.	Clinical, sports
Feetme–Health [61]	Insole with inertial sensor analysis and plantar pressure point for clinical-grade measurement of spatiotemporal variables of gait.	Clinical
GAITRite [59]	Gait analysis mat, leader in analysis for spatiotemporal variables of the gait cycle.	Clinical, academic
P-Walk [62]	Mat that measures static balance variables through the acquisition of postures and control of the center of mass and spatiotemporal variables of the gait cycle.	Clinical, academic

Table 3.
Technological systems to assess motor impairments using plantar pressures in post-stroke patients.

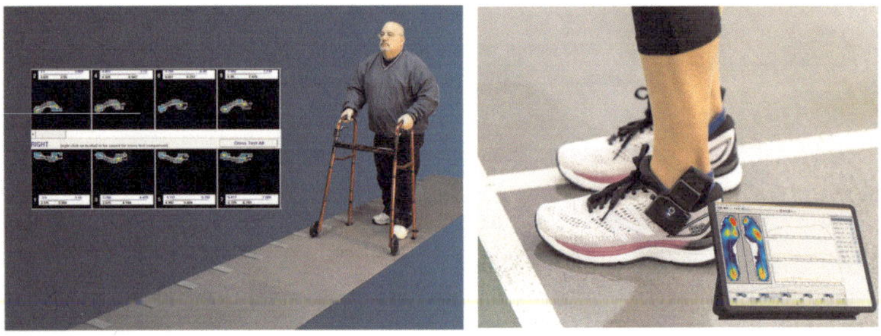

Figure 5.
Pressure-based systems to analyze gait and posture. From left to right: GAITRite and Xsensor. Images obtained from the official website of Xsensor [58] and GAITRite [59].

5.2 Technological systems for post-stroke patients rehabilitation

As mentioned at the beginning of this section, the technological tools for the treatment of post-stroke subjects seek to reduce the impact of the disabling condition to improve the quality of life of the patient through rehabilitation therapies to train or adapt the lost function.

From this perspective, the development of serious games for rehabilitation has taken on great importance in the treatment since, they make patients hooked on their treatment, avoiding problems associated with early abandonment from their therapies. Systems that use interactive platforms such as the famous Kinect (camera system) [63] and Nintendo Wii (multisensory system with inertial control and pressure platform) [64] started a massive adoption in the field of game development to support the rehabilitation. However, although they continue to be used in clinical settings for interactive treatment, these technologies are no longer commercially available and are obsolete.

Because of the great technological advance in animation and graphic processing systems, serious games for immersive or semi-immersive rehabilitation using virtual reality helmets (HTC-vive, Oculus, among others) have allowed to establish an environment that mimics in controlled conditions in the daily life of people in order to train typical activities such as brushing teeth, cooking and eating in a safe environment [65]. Also, semi-immersive elements have made it possible to instrumentalize the highly used mirror movement test to increase patients' perception of movement. All these systems that support the mobility of the upper and lower extremities allow the development of augmented reality environments or interactive systems that enrich the experience of the patient and provide more information about the patient's condition [66]. Some commercial rehabilitation options include Tyromotion's PABLO (interactive upper extremity therapy), TYMO (interactive system for balance and coordination training), and DIEGO (interactive arm and shoulder rehabilitation) systems (**Figure 6**) [67].

Leaving aside the treatment systems and focusing on systems that have the potential to be used in everyday life, functional electrical stimulation tools (FES) appear, which correspond to systems that, through the injection of controlled electrical pulses, allow to recover the mobility of limbs, improving grip in upper limb cases and improving gait in case of foot drop stimulators. Although upper limb stimulators have not yet become widespread, in the literature, there is great evidence of efforts by researchers to generate alternatives to train or regain mobility of the arms and hands. Alternatively, and more commonly, there are electronic orthoses for droop foot, where by means of a system that allows the generation of controlled pulses from the detection of gait cycle events, the control of dorsiflexion can be recovered in post-stroke patients [68]. Commercial examples are SmartFES, XFT-2001, ODFS Pace, among others (**Figure 7**) [68–70].

On the other hand, health professionals and the scientific community have developed alternatives to treat post-stroke who, due to different factors such as economical, geographical, physical, and/or environmental, are unable to attend rehabilitation centers. The need for the above has increased as a result of the recent COVID-19

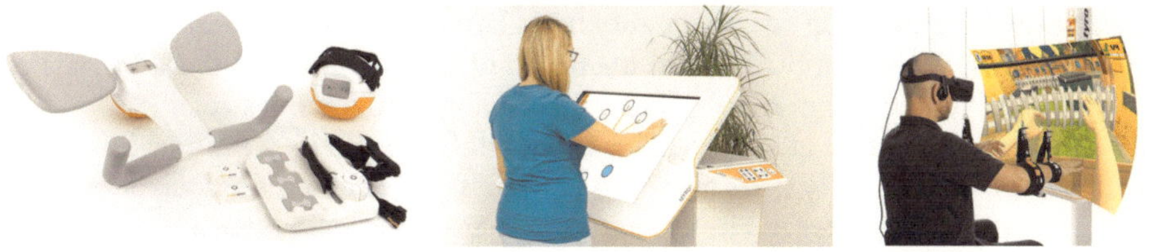

Figure 6.
Interactive rehabilitation systems developed from Tyromotion. From left to right: PABLO, TYMO, and DIEGO. Images obtained from the official website of Tyromotion [67].

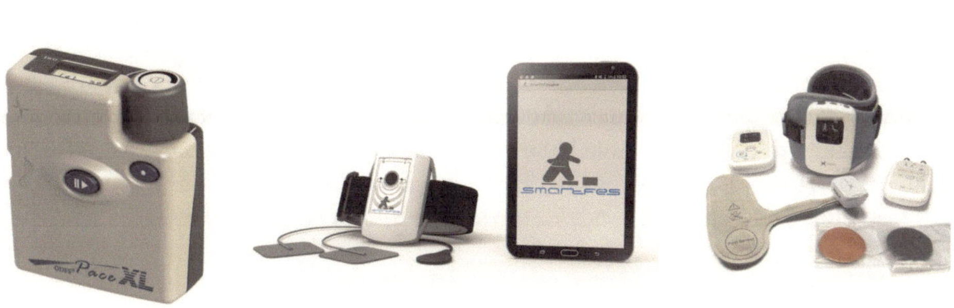

Figure 7.
Functional electrical stimulation systems commercially available. From left to right: ODFS pace, SmartFES, and XFT-2001. Images obtained from the official website of SmartFES [68], XFT-2001 [69], and Odstock [70].

pandemic that incorporates post-stroke people as a population at risk [71]. Regarding this, different types of treatment that use technology to rehabilitate communication skills [72], upper limb rehabilitation, and/or remote activities of daily living have been evaluated, proving to be almost as effective as face-to-face treatments. Although there is a lack of information on the cost-effectiveness relationship with respect to traditional treatments, it is evident that the role of telerehabilitation is of vital importance in rural areas or in health emergencies where patients do not have access to opportune care or monitoring of their condition [73, 74].

In this section, some tools typically used for the evaluation and treatment of post-stroke patients are mentioned. However, the intention is to provide a general overview of the systems most used internationally, existing alternatives that improve their proposal in terms of accessibility and costs.

6. Conclusion

Stroke generates primary and secondary impairments that reduce the functional capacity of these patients, leading to less functional independence and quality of life. One of the main impairments associated with this population is impaired balance, both static and dynamic. This impairment in particular generates a great impact on the dysfunction of activities of daily living and main transfers such as bipedal sedentary transfer and gait. Moreover, in this pathology, 14–65% of individuals fall at least once in the hospital, and between 37 and 73% suffer falls in the next 6 months after discharge [75].

Specifically, people with stroke are at increased risk of fall-related fractures. Other adverse consequences may include fear of falling with subsequent reduction in activity, de-conditioning, and increased risk of falls. Bower et al. state that it has recently been shown that the identification of movement and balance variables, for example by measuring walking speed, application of the timed up and go test, and the Berg Balance Scale, have been shown to be strong predictors of fall risk following stroke [8].

However, as mentioned above, there are some deficiencies in the clinical tests and scales, since they fail to fully determine the variables and problems associated with balance impairment. The use of clinical scales and tests, associated with the use of technologies, could allow the adequate assessment of each of the limitations in static and dynamic balance during the different transfers performed by people with sequelae of stroke.

In this chapter, we have presented a list of alternatives to treat and evaluate the stroke patient in all phases of treatment, providing plenty of evidence of systems for movement analysis and treatment, especially useful for the treating professional, and of highly technological elements to improve adherence to rehabilitation therapies.

Finally, it is important to highlight that a specific assessment of the impairments that contribute to an unfavorable balance in subjects with stroke is necessary for each rehabilitation process, as well as the early incorporation of functional therapeutic activities aimed at their recovery and the prevention of the risk of falls.

Acknowledgements

This work was supported by the Vice-rectory for research and development (VRID) of the Universidad de Concepción: “Clinical validation of a human motion analysis system based on inertial measurement sensors in a Chilean population at risk of falls" [Cod.- 220.092.003-M].

Conflict of interest

Pablo Aqueveque, Britam Gómez and Francisco Saavedra were developers of SmartFES and QMUV devices. The remaining authors have no conflicts of interest to declare.

Author details

Paulina Ortega-Bastidas[1,2*], Britam Gómez[3], Karen Barriga[1], Francisco Saavedra[3] and Pablo Aqueveque[3]

1 Faculty of Medicine, Kinesiology Department, Universidad de Concepción, Concepción, Chile

2 Health Sciences PhD Programme, Universidad Rey Juan Carlos, Madrid, Spain

3 Faculty of Engineering, Electrical Engineering Department, Universidad de Concepción, Concepción, Chile

*Address all correspondence to: portegab@udec.cl

References

[1] Li J, Zhong D, Ye J, et al. Rehabilitation for balance impairment in patients after stroke: A protocol of a systematic review and network meta-analysis. BMJ Open. 2019;**9**:e026844. DOI: 10.1136/bmjopen-2018-026844

[2] Shumway-Cook A, Woollacott M. Control Motor de la Investigación a la práctica Clínica. 5th ed. Alphen aan den Rijn, Netherlands: Wolter Kluwer; 2017. pp. 228-229

[3] Cano de La Cuerda R, Piédrola M, Miangolarra P. Control y Aprendizaje Motor. Fundamentos, desarrollo y reeducación del movimiento humano. Panamericana. 2017

[4] Horak FB. Postural Orientation and equilibruim: What do we need to know about neural control of balance to prevent falls? Age and Ageing. 2006; **35–S2**:ii7-ii11. DOI: 10.1093/ageing/afl077

[5] Cano de la Cuerda R, Callado Vasquez S. Neurorrehabilitación, Métodos específicos de valoración y tratamiento. Panamericana. 2012

[6] Winstein CJ et al. Guidelines for adult stroke rehabilitation and recovery. Stroke. 2016;**47**:e98-e169. DOI: 10.1161/STR.0000000000000098

[7] Bower KJ, McGinley JL, Miller KJ, Clark RA. Instrumented static and dynamic balance assessment after stroke using Wii Balance Boards: reliability and association with clinical tests. PloS One. 2014;**9**(12):e115282. DOI: 10.1371/journal.pone.0115282

[8] Bower K et al. Dynamic balance and instrumented gait variables are independent predictor of falls following stroke. Journal of NeuroEngineering and Rehabilitation. 2019;**16**:3. DOI: 10.1186/s12984-018-0478-4

[9] Goh H-T et al. Falls and Fear of Falling after Stroke: A case-control study. PM & R : The Journal of Injury, Function, and Rehabilitation. 2016;**8**: 1173-1180

[10] Merchant RA et al. Relationship between fear of falling, fear related activity, restriction, frailty and sarcopenia. Journal of the American Geriatrics Society. 2020;**68**:2602-2608. DOI: 10.1111/jgs.16719

[11] Boukadida A, Piotte F, Dehail P, Nadeau S. Determinant of sit-to-stand tasks in individual with hemiparesis post stroke: A review. Annals of Physical and Rehabilitation Medicine. 2015;**58**: 167-172. DOI: 10.1016/j.rehab.2015.04.007

[12] Beyaert C, Vasa R, Frykberg GE. Gait post-stroke: Pathophysiology and rehabilitation strategies. Clinical Neurophysiology. 2015;**45**:335-355

[13] Raine S, Meadows L, Lynch-Ellerington M. Bobath Concept. Theory and Clinical Practice in Neurological Rehabilitation. New York: Wiley-Blackwell; 2009. p. 83, 84, 117

[14] Chen HB, Wei TS, Chang LW. Postural Influence strategies and sitting impact forces in stroke patients. Gait and Posture. 2010;**32**:576-580. DOI: 10.1016/j.gaitpost.2010.08.005

[15] Van Bladel A, Kilinc O, De Ridder R, Kılınc M. Trunk and lower extremity biomechanics during sit-to-stand activity after stroke. Gait and Posture. 2021;**90**:280. DOI: 10.1016/j.gaitpost.2021.09.145

[16] Carr J, Seperd R. Rehabilitación en el paciente con Ictus, recomendaciones para optimizar las habilidades motoras. Amsterdam, Netherlands: Elsevier España; 2004

[17] Perry J. Gait Analysis, Normal and Pathological Function. West Deptford, NJ: Slack Incorporated; 1992

[18] Dickstein R. Rehabilitation of Gait Speed After Stroke: A critical review of intervention approaches. Neurorehabilitation and Neural Repair. 2008;**22**(6). DOI: 10.1177/1545968308315997

[19] Wang Y, Mukaino M, Otsuka K, Otaka H, et al. Gait characteristics of post-stroke hemiparetic patients with different walking speeds. International Journal of Rehabilitation Research. 2020; **43**:69-75. DOI: 10.1097/MRR.0000000000000391

[20] Wonsetler E, Bowden M. A systematic review of mechanisms of gait speed post stroke. Part 1: Spatiotemporal parameter and asymmetry ratios. Topics in Stroke Rehabilitation. 2017;**24**(6): 435-446. DOI: 10.1080/10749357.2017.1285746

[21] Stein J, Harvey R, Macko R, Winstein C, Zorowitz R. Stroke Recovery and Rehabilitation. New York: Demos Medical Publishing; 2009

[22] Hugues A, Di Marco J, Ribault S, Ardaillon H, Janiaud P, Xue Y, et al. Limited evidence of physical therapy on balance after stroke: A systematic review and meta-analysis. PLoS One. 2019; **14**(8):e0221700. DOI: 10.1371/journal.pone.0221700

[23] Van Duijnhoven H, Heeren A, Peters M, Veerbeck J, Kwakkel G, et al. Effects of exercise therapy on balance capacity on chronic stroke. Stroke. 2016;**47**: 2603-2610. DOI: 10.1161/STROKEAHA.116.013839

[24] Silva A, Sousa AS, Pinheiro R, Ferraz J, Tavares JM, Santos R, et al. Activation timing of soleus and tibialis anterior muscles during sit-to-stand and stand-to-sit in post-stroke vs. healthy subjects. Somatosensory & Motor Research. 2013; **30**(1):48-55. DOI: 10.3109/08990220.2012.754755

[25] Brière A, Nadeau S, Lauziére S, Gravel D. Perception of weight—Bearing and Effort distribution during sit-to-stand in individuals post-stroke. Perceptual & Motor Skills: Motor Skills & Ergonomic. 2013;**117**(1):166-181

[26] Balandan B. Gait Disturbance in Patients with Stroke. PM & R. 2014;**6**: 635-642. DOI: 10.1016/j.pmrj.2013.12.017

[27] Park SH. Tools for assessing fall risk in the elderly: A systematic review and meta-analysis. Aging Clinical and Experimental Research. 2018;**30**:1-16

[28] Lin Q, Zheng Y, Lian P, Guo Y, Huang H, Luo Z, et al. Quantitative static and dynamic assessment of balance control in stroke patients. Journal of Visualized Experiments. 2020;**159**: e60884. DOI: 10.3791/60884

[29] Pickenbrock H, Diel A, Zpaf A. A comparison between the static balance test and the Berg Balance Scale: Validity, reliability, and comparative resource use. Clinical Rehabilitation. 2016;**30**(3). 288-293. DOI: 10.1177/0269215515578297

[30] Neuls PD, Clark TL, Van Heuklon NC, Proctor JE, Kilker BJ, et al. Usefulness of the berg balance scale to predict falls in the elderly. Journal of Geriatric Physical Therapy. 2011;**34**: 3-10

[31] Donoghue D, Stokes E. How much change is true change. The minimum detectable change of the berg balance scale in elderly people. Journal of Rehabilitation Medicine. 2009;**41**:343-346

[32] Lusardi MM. Functional performance in community living older adults. Journal of Geriatric Physical Therapy. 2004;**26**(3):14-22

[33] Zasadzka E, Borowicz AM, Roszak M, Pawlaczyk M. Assessment of the risk of falling with the use of timed up and go test in the elderly with lower extremity osteoarthritis. Clinical Interventions in Aging. 2015;**10**:1289

[34] Persson CU, Danielsson A, Sunnerhagen KS, Grimby-Ekman A, Hansson PO. Timed Up and Go as a measure for longitudinal change in mobility after stroke–Postural Stroke Study in Gothenburg (POSTGOT). Journal of Neuroengineering and Rehabilitation. 2014;**11**:83

[35] Nguyen H, Lebel K, Boissy P, Bogard S, Goubault E, Duval C. Auto detection and segmentation of daily living activities during a timed up and go task in people with Parkinson's disease using multiple inertial sensors. Journal of Neuroengineering and Rehabilitation. 2017;**14**:26

[36] Podsiadlo D, Richardson S. The timed Up and Go: A test of basic functional mobility for frail elderly persons. Journal of the American Geriatrics Society. 1991;**39**:142-148

[37] Mancilla E. Rendimiento en las pruebas Timed up and Go y Estación Unipodal en AM chileno entre 60 y 89 años. Revista medica de Chile. 2015;**143**: 39-46

[38] Flansbjer U. Realiability of gait performance tests in men and women with hemiparesis after stroke. Journal of Rehabilitation Medicine. 2005;**37**:75-82

[39] Hafsteinsdóttir T. Clinimetric properties of the timed up and go test for patients with stroke: A systematic review. Topics in Stroke Rehabilitation. 2014;**21**(3):197-210

[40] Barry E, Galvin R, Keogh C, Horgan F, Fahey T. Is the timed up and go test a useful predictor of risk of falls in community dwelling older adults: A systematic review and meta-analysis. BMC Geriatrics. 2014;**14**:14

[41] Middleton A, Lusardi M. Walking sped: The functional vital sign. Journal of Aging and Physical Activity. 2015;**23**(2): 314-322

[42] Tysson S, Connel L. The psychometric properties and clinical utility of measures of walking and mobility in neurological conditions. A systematic review. Clinical Rehabilitation. 2009;**23**:1018-1033

[43] Perry J, Garret M, Gronley JK, Mulroy SJ. Classification of waling handicap in the stroke population. Stroke. 1995;**26**(6):982-989

[44] Shirley Ryan—Abilitylab. Available from: https://www.sralab.org/ [Accessed: July 19, 2021]

[45] Tsang C et al. Psychometric properties of the mini-balance evaluation systems test (Mini-BESTest) in community-dwelling individuals whit chronic stroke. Physical Therapy. 2013; **93**:1102-1115

[46] Horak F, Wrisley D, Frank J. The balance evaluation systems test (BESTest) to differentiate balances defitics. Physical Therapy. 2009;**89**(5): 484-498. DOI: 10.2522/ptj.20080071

[47] Di Carlo S et al. The mini-BESTest: A review of psychometric properties. International Journal of Rehabilitation Research. 2016;**39**:97-105

[48] Hawyama K, Kawakami M, Otsuka T. Effect of core stability training on trunk function, standing balance, and mobility in Stroke patients: A randomized controlled trial. Neurorehabilitation and Neural Repair. 2017;**31**(3):240-249. DOI: 10.1177/1545968316675431

[49] Timmermans AA, Seelen HA, Willmann RD, Kingma H. Technology-assisted training of arm-hand skills in stroke: Concepts on reacquisition of motor control and therapist guidelines for rehabilitation technology design. Journal of Neuroengineering and Rehabilitation. 2009;**6**(1):1-18

[50] Optitrack System. Available from: https://optitrack.com/ [Accessed: November 5, 2021]

[51] G-Walk System. Available from: https://www.btsbioengineering.com/es/products/g-walk/ [Accessed: November 10, 2021]

[52] Mobility Lab System. Available from: https://apdm.com/mobility/ [Accessed: November 15, 2021]

[53] QMUV Inertial System. Available from: https://qmuv.cl/ [Accessed: November 1, 2021]

[54] Vicon System. Available from: https://www.vicon.com/ [Accessed: November 3, 2021]

[55] MTw Axinda System. Available from: https://www.xsens.com/products/mtw-awinda [Accessed: November 2, 2021]

[56] Perception Neuron Pro System. Available from: https://neuronmocap.com/ [Accessed: October 28, 2021]

[57] Ultium Motion System. Available from: https://www.noraxon.com/our-products/ultium-motion/ [Accessed: November 7, 2021]

[58] Xsensor Insole System. Available from: https://es.xsensor.com/ [Accessed: November 5, 2021]

[59] GAITRite Mat System. Available from: https://www.gaitrite.com/ [Accessed: November 7, 2021]

[60] Moticon Insole System. Available from: https://moticon.com/ [Accessed: November 6, 2021]

[61] Feetme–Health Insole System. Available from: https://feetmehealth.com/insoles/ [Accessed: November 6, 2021]

[62] P-Walk Mat System. Available from: https://www.btsbioengineering.com/products/p-walk/ [Accessed: November 7, 2021]

[63] Ferreira D, Oliveira R, Postolache O. Physical rehabilitation based on kinect serious games. In: Eleventh International Conference on Sensing Technology (ICST). New York: IEEE; 2017. pp. 1-6

[64] Dos Santos LRA, Carregosa AA, Masruha MR, Dos Santos PA, Coêlho MLDS, Ferraz DD, et al. The use of nintendo wii in the rehabilitation of poststroke patients: A systematic review. Journal of Stroke and Cerebrovascular Diseases. 2015;**24**(10):2298-2305

[65] Wade E, Winstein CJ. Virtual reality and robotics for stroke rehabilitation: Where do we go from here? Topics in Stroke Rehabilitation. 2011;**18**(6):685-700

[66] Loureiro RC, Harwin WS, Nagai K, Johnson M. Advances in upper limb stroke rehabilitation: A technology push. Medical and Biological Engineering and Computing. 2011;**49**(10):1103-1118

[67] Tyromotion Products. Available from: https://tyromotion.com/en/product-overview/ [Accessed: November 20, 2021]

[68] Aqueveque P, Ortega P, Pino E, Saavedra F, Germany E, Gómez B. After stroke movement impairments: A review of current technologies for rehabilitation. Physical Disabilities-Therapeutic Implications. 2017;**10**:95-116

[69] SmartFES System. Available from: http://smartfes.cl/ [Accessed: November 12, 2021]

[70] Odstock System. Available from: https://odstockmedical.com/prod-category/stimulators/ [Accessed: November 12, 2021]

[71] Chang, M. C., and Boudier-Revéret, M. (2020). Usefulness of Telerehabilitation for Stroke Patients during the COVID-19 Pandemic. American Journal of Physical Medicine and Rehabilitation 997 p 582 doi: 10.1097/PHM.0000000000001468

[72] Agostini M, Garzon M, Benavides-Varela S, De Pellegrin S, Bencini G, Rossi G, et al. Telerehabilitation in poststroke anomia. BioMed Research International. 2014;**2014**:1-6. DOI: 10.1155/2014/706909

[73] Johansson T, Wild C. Telerehabilitation in stroke care—A systematic review. Journal of Telemedicine and Telecare. 2011;**17**(1):1-6. DOI: 10.1258/jtt.2010.100105

[74] Laver KE, Adey-Wakeling Z, Crotty M, Lannin NA, George S, Sherrington C. Telerehabilitation services for stroke. Cochrane Database of Systematic Reviews. 2020;**1**

[75] Beghi E, Gervasoni E, Pupillo E, Bianchi E, Montesano A, Aprile I, et al. Prediction of falls in subjects suffering from parkinson disease, multiple sclerosis, and stroke. Archives of Physical Medicine and Rehabilitation. 2018;**99**:641-651. DOI: 10.1016/j.ampr.2017.10.009

Section 2

Post-Stroke Rehabilitation: Risk Factors

Chapter 4

Cultural Beliefs and Psychosocial Stress Are Unseen Potential Predisposing Factors for Stroke in Sub-Saharan Africa: Reality for Post-Stroke Rehabilitation

Polycarp Umunna Nwoha, Florence Osita Okoro, Emmanuel Chukwudi Nwoha, Augustine Obi, Chidinma Oluchi Nwoha, Iyanu Ayoola, Nkeiru Christiana Ogoko, Peace Ngozi Nwoha, Anna Idaguko, Catherine Wali, Nnenna Chinagozi-Amanze and Ifeoma H. Nwoha-Okpara

Abstract

This work considered post-stroke rehabilitation in sub-Saharan Africa, referencing psychosocial stress and wrongful cultural beliefs. Stroke, a neurological disease preventable by lifestyle changes, is increasing at, particularly in sub-Saharan Africa (SSA). First-ever stroke cases stand the risk of a second, which could be fatal; hence the need for review of post-stroke rehabilitation strategies. In our work on survivors, we noted that most established risk factors do not necessarily apply in SSA. Of the 10 risk factors studied, hypertension was the commonest reported. In our study of 149 survivors in Nigeria, 73.1% suffered from hypertension; only 53.7% were aware of their hypertensive status before stroke incidence. When asked about risk factors, 19.4% mentioned hypertension, 0.7% diabetes mellitus but 13.1% psychological stress, and 13.4% spiritual attack/diabolical; 39.6% had no idea what caused stroke. The findings show the role hypertension, psychological stress and cultural ignorance play in fueling stroke in SSA. Further, 97.3% of survivors were married, 65.1% had 5 to 8 children, engaged in sedentary occupations, trading, farming, civil service, occupations also prone to economic woes in Nigeria. Commonest age of survivors was 60 to 75 years; a period of very stressful life in Nigeria. All these culminate to sustained psychosocial pressures, hypertension and stroke. There is urgent need to reduce psychosocial pressures, correct wrongful cultural beliefs, especially among survivors in sub-Saharan Africa. The strength of this work lies in the observation of lack of awareness and community screening as the most pronounced common variable among the survivors. The place of herbal medicine in post-stroke rehabilitation should be recognised. Of the 117 survivors who visited Bebe Herbal Centre for management, 99.1% were satisfied; 67.5% of them had satisfactory recovery in less than 1 month. Introduction of physiotherapy in Herbal centres would speed up recovery.

Keywords: psychosocial stress, family pressure, occupational pressure, herbal treatment, cultural beliefs, stroke awareness

1. Introduction

Stroke is a menace to the society. All over the world, it affects countless number of people, as much as 16 million people per year [1]. Out of this number, 5.7 million die, and the rest becomes disabled for a long period, even for life. It is the second most common cause of death worldwide, after ischaemic heart disease [2–4]. The impact of stroke is mostly felt in low and middle income countries. About 85% of all stroke deaths are registered in low and middle income countries, which also account for 87% of total losses due to stroke in terms disability-adjusted life years calculated worldwide per year [2]. As the burden of stroke has shifted to the developing world, currently two-thirds of stroke mortality cases occur in sub-Saharan Africa (SSA), [2–4]. This is sad because this is the same region that poverty, malnutrition and communicable diseases also exert their greatest toll [5]. The unfortunate thing is that while the proportion of stroke is decreasing in the developed world, it is rising alarmingly in the under-developed world [6]. The World Health has predicted that by the year 2030, majority (80%) of stroke cases would be in the low-income and middle-income countries. Africa, in particular, records some of the highest rates of stroke worldwide, with an annual stroke incidence rate up to 316 per 100,000, prevalence rate up to 1460 per 100,000 and three-year fatality rate up to 84% [7–10]. In Africa, stroke accounts for 4–9% of deaths and between 6.5–41% of neurological admissions, as reported in hospital-based studies [11, 12]. This is not only alarming, it is frightening; and should concern all of us. Two-thirds of stroke cases worldwide occur in SSA [13]. It is, therefore, clear that sub-Saharan Africa has become the epicentre of stroke in the world, calling for strong sustained efforts to reduce the incidence of stroke in the region. This reality should provoke increased attention to stroke issues in the world, especially in the low- and middle-income countries, in order to reverse the trend. In doing this, we must firstly identify the real problems associated with stroke in the region. For post-stroke rehabilitation effort to be effective and set goals of preventing second stroke achieved, it is important to focus attention on the real factors that predispose to stoke in the region. All factors should be taken into account, including the role of herbal centres and cultural beliefs, which have long been neglected. Great effort should be focused in reducing stroke occurrence in sub-Saharan Africa, because of the cumulative positive effect it would have on stroke reduction the world over. Fortunately and surprisingly, stroke is the most preventable of all neurological diseases as many of its risk factors, such as hypertension, high cholesterol, diabetes, and smoking can be prevented either through healthy lifestyle choices or by medication [14, 15]. In sub-Saharan Africa, therefore, psychosocial pressures and cultural beliefs should be given due attention, especially in post-stroke rehabilitation programmes.

2. Demographic study

This section discusses majorly the demographic features of 149 stroke survivors who visited Bebe Herbal Centre located in Umunomo Ihitteafoukwu, Ahiazu Mbaise, Imo state, Nigeria, for treatment and their import on stroke issues in sub-Saharan Africa. In the study [16] (**Tables 1–3**), it was noted that 97.3% of survivors were married while 2.7% were single. What this means is that being married is a potential source of pressure, especially for the low-income group. It was also reported that 65.1% of those married had 5 to 8 children, further strengthening our

Age (years)	Frequency n (%)		Total
	Gender		
	Male	Female	
<40	3 (2.0)	3 (2.0)	6 (4.0)
40–44	2 (1.3)	0 (0.0)	2 (1.3)
45–49	3 (2.0)	2 (1.3)	5 (3.4)
50–54	7 (4.7)	12 (8.1)	19 (12.8)
55–59	10 (6.7)	9 (6.0)	19 (12.8)
60–64	13 (8.7)	8 (5.4)	21 (14.1)
65–69	7 (4.7)	9 (6.0)	16 (10.7)
70–74	27 (8.1)	9 (6.0)	36 (24.2)
75–79	10 (6.7)	7 (4.7)	17 (11.4)
80+	6 (4.0)	2 (1.3)	8 (5.4)
Side affected			
Left	52 (34.9)	32 (21.5)	84 (56.4)
Right	36 (24.2)	29 (19.5)	65 (43.6)
Educational attainment			
Illiterate	0 (0)	4 (2.7)	4 (2.7)
Primary	42 (28.2)	38 (25.5)	80 (53.7)
Secondary	26 (17.4)	14 (9.4)	40 (26.8)
Tertiary	20 (13.4)	5 (3.4)	25 (16.8)
Occupation			
Unemployed	0 (0)	1 (1.6)	1 (1.6)
Trading	19 (12.8)	23 (15.4)	42 (28.2)
Artisan	30 (20.1)	11 (7.4)	41 (27.5)
Farming	12 (8.1)	21 (14.1)	33 (22.1)
Civil servant	27 (18.1)	5 (3.4)	32 (21.5)

Nwoha et al. [16].

Table 1.
Distribution of parameters among male and female stroke survivors (n = 149).

Variable	<45 years	45-64 years	≥65 years	Total
Gender				
Male	5 (3.4)	32 (21.5)	58 (38.9)	95 (63.8)
Female	4 (2.6)	28 (18.8)	22 (14.8)	54 (36.2)
Marital status				
Married	6 (4.0)	60 (40.3)	79 (53.0)	145 (97.3)
Single	3 (2.0)	1 (0.7)	0 (0)	4 (2.7)
Number of children				
1–4	5 (3.4)	21 (14.1)	12 (8.1)	38 (2.5)
5–8	0 (0)	37 (24.8)	60 (40.3)	97 (65.1)
>8	1 (0.7)	4 (2.7)	9 (6.0)	14 (9.3)
Highest educational level				
Illiterate	0 (0)	1 (0.7)	3 (2.0)	4 (2.7)
Primary	2 (1.3)	28 (18.7)	51 (34.0)	81 (54.0)
Secondary	4 (2.7)	19 (12.7)	11 (7.3)	34 (22.7)
Tertiary	3 (2.0)	14 (9.3)	13 (8.7)	30 (20.0)
Occupation				
Unemployed	1 (0.7)	2 (1.3)	1 (0.7)	4 (2.7)
Civil servants	2 (1.3)	15 (10.1)	15 (10.1)	32 (21.5)
Artisans	1 (0.7)	6 (4.0)	14 (9.4)	21 (14.1)
Traders	5 (3.3)	31 (20.8)	22 (14.7)	58 (38.9)
Farmers	0 (0)	10 (6.7)	24 (16.1)	34 (22.8)
Season of the year				
Nov.–April (Dry)	6 (4.0)	46 (30.9)	52 (34.9)	104 (69.8)
May–October (Wet)	3 (2.0)	16 (10.7)	26 (17.4)	45 (30.2)

Nwoha et al. [16].

Table 2.
Distribution of size of variables relative to age (year) of respondents (frequency, percentage).

position that in SSA, having large families is potentially a big source of psychosocial pressure, which could lead to hypertension and eventual stroke. The reason is because of the low income capacity of most of these families in the region. Inability to cater for one's family poses serious psychosocial pressure; and the larger the family, the more the pressure on parents and guardians. Cooper et al. [17] noted in their work that high blood pressure is the foundation of epidaemic cardiovascular diseases in Africa. To prevent a stroke event, especially for survivors, there is need to reduce avoidable pressures from families, for example, by limiting the number of children one caters for. Government should also help by providing social welfare programmes, including subsidising health and education for her low-income citizens. These, if done, will take a lot of pressure off low-income large families.

One's occupation in sub-Saharan Africa could also be a source of psychosocial pressure. In our work, we noted that people most commonly affected by stroke were traders (38.9%) followed by farmers and civil servants, in that order, 22.8% and

Variables	Male	Female	X^2	Df	P
	n (%)	n (%)			
Age group (yrs)			**12.04**	**9**	**0.211**
<45	6 (4.0)	3 (2.0)			
45-49	3 (2.0)	2 (1.3)			
50-54	6 (4.0)	12 (8.1)			
55-59	9 (6.0)	9 (6.0)			
60-64	14 (9.4)	8 (5.4)			
65-69	7 (4.7)	9 (6.0)			
70-74	27 (18.1)	9 (6.0)			
75-79	10 (6.7)	7 (4.7)			
≥80	6 (4.0)	2 (1.3)			
Education			**12.31**	**3**	**0.006**
Primary school	41 (27.5)	38 (25.5)			
Secondary schol	25 (16.8)	14 (9.4)			
Tertiary school	19 (12.8)	5 (3.4)			
No school	3 (2.0)	4 (2.7)			
Occupation			**23.65**	**4**	**0.001**
Unemployed	4 (2.7)	1 (0.7)			
Trader	18 (12.1)	23 (15.4)			
Artisan	29 (19.5)	11 (7.4)			
Farmer	11 (7.4)	21 (14.1)			
Civil servant	26 (17.4)	5 (3.4)			
Side body affected			**0.403**	**3**	**0.296**
Left	52 (34.9)	32 (21.5)			
Right	36 (24.2)	29 (19.5)			
Number of children			**1.146**	**2**	**0.96**
No child	4 (2.7)	3 (2.0)			
01-Apr	19 (12.8)	16 (10.7)			
05-Aug	56 (37.6)	35 (23.5)			
Above 8	9 (6.0)	7 (4.7)			

Nwoha et al. [16].

Table 3.
Descriptive characteristic of the survivors and person's chi-squared test between male and female.

21.5% respectively. Artisans were not much affected (14.1%) while the unemployed were barely affected (2.7%). Pearson's chi-squared test (**Table 3**) shows evidence of strong association between education, and occupation and gender of stroke survivors. Education had strong significant association ($X2 = 12.31$; $df = 3$, $p < .006$). More men than women had primary education (27.5% vs. 25.5%), secondary education (16.8% vs. 9.4%) and tertiary education (12.8% vs. 3.4%). Occupation

Variables	Male (n, %)	Female (n, %)	χ^2	df	p
Hypertension			**3.68**	3	**0.296**
Aware before stroke	44 (29.5)	36 (24.2)			
Aware after stroke	16 (10.7)	13 (8.7)			
No knowledge	12 (8.1)	3 (2.0)			
Not hypertensive	16 (10.7)	9 (6.0)			
Diabetes mellitus			**.082**	2	**0.960**
Yes, diabetic	24 (16.1)	16 (10.7)			
No knowledge	17 (11.4)	11 (7.4)			
Not diabetic	47 (31.5)	34 (22.8)			
Alcohol intake			**24.23**	1	**0.001**
Yes	67 (45.0)	21 (14.1)			
Never	21 (14.1)	40 (26.8)			
Cigarette smoking			**9.823**	1	**0.001**
Yes	37 (24.8)	10 (6.7)			
Never	51 (34.2)	51 (34.2)			

Table 4.
Stroke risk factors suffered/encountered by survivors and Pearson's chi-squared test of association with gender.

had significant strong association with gender of the stroke survivors (X2 = 23.65; df = 4; p < .001) with more men than women being unemployed (2.7% vs. 0.7%), being artisans (19.5% vs. 3.4%) and civil servants (17.4% vs. 3.4%) while women more than men were traders (15.4% vs. 12.1%) and farmers (14.1% vs. 7.4%). By the age bracket indicated, most people in these professions would have retired from active service and be faced with the burden of lower income generation for their numerous bourgeoning responsibilities, leading to increased psychosocial pressure and hypertension. We also noted that those with primary education only were highest among the stroke survivors [53.7%], followed by secondary education and tertiary. The higher the educational level, the higher the tendency for better income and also the likelihood of better awareness of stroke risk factors. These add up to better lifestyle and low stroke incidence for those with higher education. Individuals, particularly the first-stroke ones, should be aware of these factors that fuel stroke via psychosocial pressure and hypertension. Socioeconomic status has long been identified as a risk factor for hypertension [18]. In a meta-analysis, multiple indicators of socioeconomic status (i.e., income, occupation, and education) were associated with an increased risk of hypertension. It was suggested that working conditions induce stress that is associated with increased risk of hypertension [18]. We also noted in our work that very few stroke cases were below 40 years of age while the most were between 60 and 74 years, the age group when family pressures are highest in sub-Saharan Africa. High levels of anxiety and depressive symptoms are common in adults, often comorbid with chronic illnesses such as hypertension and can have deleterious effects on individual health and quality of life. A meta-analysis of prospective studies found that depressive symptoms predict a 42% increased risk of hypertension [19]. Similarly a meta-analysis of prospective studies fund that anxiety symptoms were independent risk factor for hypertension [20].

Stressors linked with unemployment, underemployment, job conflict, or financial strain due to low wages may lead to hypertension. An explanation for this was provided by Everson-Rose et al. [21] who noted that psychosocial factors, such as hostility and job strain, are associated with higher circulating levels of catecholamines, higher cortisol levels, and increased blood pressure over time. Psychosocial factors that induce emotional stress can evoke a physiological response mediated in part by activation of the sympathetic nervous system, inflammation, and the hypothalamic–pituitary–adrenal axis (**Table 4**) [22, 23].

3. Risk factors

There are traditional risk factors for stroke, including hypertension, dyslipidemia, diabetes mellitus, obesity, smoking, stress (physical and emotional), sedentary lifestyle, heavy alcohol consumption, previous stroke and family history of stroke [2, 24]. Of these, hypertension is an important risk factor for a variety of health conditions, such as cardiovascular disease, stroke, and kidney failure. Hypertension is the leading risk factor for stroke and is present in nearly 1 in 3 American adults [25]. Hypertension is a pervasive problem in the United States, with approximately a third of Americans reporting being diagnosed with hypertension by their physicians or taking antihypertensive drugs [26]. It is considered the foundation for epidaemic cardiovascular diseases in African populations [17]. In Nigeria and sub-Saharan Africa, hypertension is the most important stroke risk factor [27, 28]. Growing evidence points to multiple psychological and social factors as contributors to the onset of trajectory of hypertension. It is time to understand that greater acculturation is associated with increased risk of hypertension, independent of age, gender, race/ethnicity, education, smoking, alcohol, physical activity, body mass index, and diabetes [29]. Wrong cultural beliefs do more harm than the direct risk factors.

We have greater need to educate people that hypertension is the foremost cause of stroke in sub-Saharan Africa and that psychosocial stress is the factor mostly fuelling hypertension. If we can curtail excessive and sustained psychosocial pressures and wrong cultural beliefs, we would be curtailing stroke incidence considerably. Diabetes mellitus is second causative factor for stroke in SSA but is usually accompanied by hypertension. Rarely does it alone cause stroke. Dyslipidemia (high blood cholesterol) is a third causative factor for stroke in most developed countries but rarely noted in SSA. The remaining seven traditional risk factors, namely obesity, smoking, stress (physical and mental), sedentary lifestyle, heavy alcohol consumption, previous stroke and family history of stroke are rarely recognised in sub-Saharan Africa when issues about stroke are discussed. This observation is supported by findings in our work (**Table 5**) [30] in which the commonest risk factor experienced by stroke survivors was hypertension (73.1%), followed by light alcohol consumption (59.1%), smoking (31.5%) and diabetes mellitus (26.7%). It is to be noted that 15 (10.1%) of survivors had no knowledge of their hypertensive status and 28 (18.8%) none of their diabetic status. No survivor ever did blood cholesterol test. When asked to state factors that could contribute to stroke, just 19.4% mentioned hypertension while insignificant number, 0.7%, each mentioned diabetes, family history, poor diet (excessive salt intake, low vegetables and fruits intake), overweight/obesity and 2.0% mentioned high alcohol consumption. Interestingly, a large number attributed stroke in this part of the world to psychosocial stress (worry) (13.5%), spiritual attack (13.4%) and usual illness (9.4%); factors that have no empirical evidence. Still a very

Variables	Male	Female	X^2	Df	P
	N, (%)	N, (%)			
Risk factors of stroke			**12.04**	**9**	**0.211**
Hypertension	20 (13.4)	9 (6.0)			
Diabetes	0 (0.0)	1 (0.7)			
Alcohol	3 (2.0)	0 (0.0)			
Family history of stroke	1 (0.7)	0 (0.0)			
Psychosocial stress	8 (5.4)	12 (8.1)			
Spiritual attack	13 (8.7)	7 (4.7)			
Normal Sickness	9 (6.0)	5 (3.4)			
Poor diet	0 (0.0)	1 (0.7)			
Overweight	0 (0.0)	1 (0.7)			
Don't know	34 (22.8)	25 (16.8)			
Advice to prevent stroke			**11.782**	**9**	**0.226**
Check blood pressure					
Pray to god	3 (2.0)	5 (3.4)			
Avoid stress/worry	7 (4.7)	6 (4.0)			
Alcohol	10 (6.7)	9 (6.0)			
Medical check-up	1 (0.7)	0 (0.0)			
Good behavior	7 (4.7)	3 (2.0)			
Avoid sugar	9 (6.0)	2 (1.3)			
Visit Bebe center	0 (0.0)	2 (1.3)			
Avoid diabolical people	1 (0.7)	0 (0.0)			
No advice to give	0 (0.0)	1 (0.7)			
	30 (20.1)	24 (16.1)			

Table 5.
Survivors idea of causes of stroke, their advice for prevention and Pearson's correlation with gender.

disturbing number (39.6%) had no idea what could cause a stroke. The aforementioned observations paint a gloomy picture of continued growth in stroke epidemic in this part of the world. If stroke survivors could be so ignorant of the cause of their stroke, then the possibility that they would engage in life-changing behaviours that would prevent future stroke is very remote. This study has strongly pointed to lack of awareness and community screening as the most pronounced common variable among the survivors. There is therefore, the strong need for awareness campaign and community screening, especially among post-stroke cases.

Attention should be focused on psychosocial stress as major contributing factor to stroke in this part of the world. We noted that a lot of things that contribute to pressures on the individual, including economic stress which comprises uncertainties in payment of salaries and allowances of workers to unemployment of breadwinners of families, social stress related to taking care of immediate and extended families, occupational stress resulting from uncertainty of daily outcome of market, farming, and artisan jobs. All of these converge to cause high blood pressure. The more these psychological and social pressures mount, the more the tendency to high blood pressure and hypertension. These economic anomalies may not obtain in developed countries but they are commonplace in the underdeveloped ones. Prior reviews have also identified a number of psychosocial indicators as potential risk factors for the onset and progression of hypertension [31]. Besides ignorance of actual risk factors for stroke, it is also revealing to note that many individuals, even those who have suffered a stroke, do not know the signs of an impending stroke. In our unpublished work on identifying stroke signs among stroke survivors, very few could identify the 3 cardinal signs of impending stroke, FAST (F for facial palsy, A for arm palsy, S for speech palsy and T for time to call stroke ambulance). There should be emphasis on stroke warning signs, comprising sudden disarthria (speech impairment), haemiparesis, facial palsy, dizziness/vertigo, parasthaesia, acute headache, and visual impairment. People, particularly first-ever stroke cases, should learn to avoid extreme emotional reaction to sudden painful situations in order to avoid sudden spike in blood pressure, which could lead to instant stroke. In our work, some stroke survivors recounted how their stroke occurred immediately they received painful sad news of sudden loss of loved ones, property or goods. Stroke survivors should learn to take life easy and not overreact to avoid the risk of a second stroke. For a disease such as a stroke with high incidence, this study is severely underpowered to draw any meaningful conclusions. More work in this area is needed to augment the present observations.

4. Stroke Management in Herbal Centre (cultural/traditional hospital)

For effective stroke prevention and post-stroke management in sub-Saharan Africa, due attention should be paid to the contribution of herbal centres in stroke management. This aspect of health delivery has been neglected for far too long. Yet traditional healing and herbal centres seem to matter a lot in stroke management in sub-Saharan Africa. Our work on satisfactory management of stroke by herbal homes, which is the first documented of such research, is quite informative [32]. In the study of 117 survivors who patronised Bebe Herbal Centre, we found that with the onset of stroke event, 72 (61.5%) went firstly to hospital before going to Bebe Centre, 25 (21.4%) went to other places, including prayer houses, before going to the Centre while 20 (17.1%) went firstly to the Centre. Regarding satisfactory recovery of the survivors, 116 (99.1%) said they had satisfactory recovery while attending Bebe Centre; and only one person (0.9%) said he had no recovery. Regarding time taken before the satisfactory recovery, 79 (67.5%) experienced it within 1 month of attending Bebe Centre while 73 (67.5%) had theirs after 1 month but under 6 months of attendance. All the seventy-two survivors (61.5%) that firstly went to hospital said they were not satisfied with treatment received in the hospitals while the remaining that did not go said hospital was not suitable for stroke management. None of the hospitals visited by the survivors was equipped with CT scan or MRI test machines. The consensus statement by the Helsingborg Conference demands computerised tomography for all patients with symptoms suggestive of stroke [33]. With CT scan and MRI test, ischaemic is differentiated from haemorrhagic stroke, and in case of ischaemic, recombinant tissue plasminogen activator (rt-PA) can be administered early enough to open up clogged arteries and allow reflow of blood to the injured cells, hence aiding quick recovery of the cells [34]. This benefit is only for patients who arrive stroke centres within 4.5 hours of stroke icthus. In our work, out of 72 (61.5%) survivors that

Variables	Male (n, %)	Female (n, %)	P
Activity at stroke onset			**0.713**
Sleeping	18 (15.4)	18 (15.4)	
Resting	24 (20.5)	22 (17.1)	
Physical activity	15 (12.8)	20 (17.1)	
1st place visited after onset			**0.247**
Hospital	35 (29.9)	37 (31.6)	
Bebe center	07 (6.0)	13 (11.1)	
Others	15 (12.8)	10 (8.5)	
Recovery time			**0.454**
<1 month	40 (34.2)	39 (33.3)	
1–3 months	12 (10.3)	12 (10.3)	
4–6 months	01 (0.9)	05 (4.3)	
>6 months	04 (3.4)	03 (2.6)	
No recovery	0	01 (0.9)	
After 6 months			
Impression Bebe Hospital (Cultural)			**0.380**
Very satisfied	19 (16.2)	13 (11.1)	
Satisfied	34 (29.1)	39 (33.3)	
Fairly satisfied	04 (03.4)	07 (6.0)	
Not satisfied	0	01 (0.9)	
Impression at Conventional Allopathic Hospital			**0.490**
Not satisfied	51 (43.6)	21 (17.9)	
Not suitable	15 (12.8)	30 (25.7)	
BP check before stroke			**0.323**
Once/week	11 (9.4)	11 (9.4)	
>Once/week	06 (5.1)	11 (9.4)	
Occasional	20 (17.1)	37 (31.5)	
None	6 (5.4)	15 (12.7)	
BP check after stroke			**0.054***
Once/week	18 (15.4)	12 (10.3)	
>once/week	20 (17.1)	36 (30.8)	
Occasional	09 (7.7)	07 (6.0)	
None	10 (8.5)	05 (4.3)	

$^{*}P < 0.05$.
Okoro et al. [32].

Table 6.
Experience of stroke survivors with hospital and Bebe Centre, Pearson's Chi-Square test of association with sex.

visited hospital first at the onset of stroke, 93.3% reached hospital within 6 hours of onset but none within 4.5 hours. Nonetheless, in the absence of CT and MRI in the hospitals visited, the survivors would not have benefitted even if they had arrived within the 4.5 hours window because of absence of neurodiagnostic machines. The above findings suggest two things namely the need for the establishment of stroke centres and units with neurodiagnostic equipment and expert personnel and the need for victims to arrive early at specialised hospitals within 4.5 hours of event. Unfortunately, only very few centers in sub-Saharan Africa have CT scan and MRI testing machines unlike in developed countries [35].

While considering factors that discourage stroke patients from seeking early hospital intervention, it should also be remembered that cultural beliefs have also become unintended setback in seeking behaviour among stroke patients in Nigeria [36]. Every ethnic group has a culture and tradition that may impact on their perception and understanding of an ailment. Stroke has been interpreted as a sign of the "gods" or "spirits" being angry [36]. Public education on risk factors will help diffuse these perceptions and hopefully increase patients being brought in for early hospital intervention in Nigeria [37], and other developing countries like Ghana [38], India [39] and even China [40]. Stroke rehabilitation services in Nigeria and most sub-Saharan Africa are limited to physiotherapy, only available in limited number of hospitals. They are rarely available outside hospital settings and certainly not in herbal homes. So there is urgent need to extend physiotherapy and other rehabilitation services to outside hospital settings, particularly to herbal homes to quicken recovery of stroke patients. The management of Bebe Centre, in our interaction, said their treatment was based purely on leaves and roots of trees and plants. If that is so, then there is the need for stroke survivors to embrace high vegetables and fruits in their diet. It is important to note the findings of Opie and Seedat [41] about risk factors for stroke in sub-Saharan Africa. They noted the impact of 6 topmost modifiable factors associated with stoke in descending order of population attributable risk (95% CI) to be hypertension 88.7%, dyslipidemia 48.2%, diabetes mellitus 22.6%, low green vegetable consumption 18.2%, stress 14.5% (**Table 6**).

5. Conclusions

In conclusions, for serious and successful post-stroke effective rehabilitation in sub-Saharan Africa, there should be dedicated and sustained awareness education of stroke risk factors and warning signs, especially targeted at stroke survivors because they are at high risk of a second stroke. The awareness education should dispel erroneous beliefs about stroke in this region, emphasising the ugly relationship between psychosocial stress and hypertension as the major fuel for stroke in sub-Saharan Africa. Government should contribute to lowering stroke incidence by establishing stroke units, equipped with CT scan, MRI imaging, experts and emergency response ambulances for stroke distress calls. High risk individuals should be taught to be aware of FAST as cardinal warning signs leading eventually to stroke. Herbal centres should be upgraded to continue to provide alternative management of stroke as most stroke survivors are comfortable with treatment received from them. This also calls for the need for stroke patients to favour vegetable and fruit diets because of high fibre content for lowering diabetes and blood pressure, and for their high anti-oxidant content for mopping up excess radicals. Community Physiotherapists should be deployed to herbal centres to teach and train survivors for better treatment outcome. Overall, people, including stroke survivors, should not overstress themselves physically and emotionally, curtailing family and occupational pressures, subjecting themselves to metabolic screening. Overall, this work, conducted in one setting, is severely underpowered to draw any meaningful conclusions. The unique contribution, however, is the observation of a relation with cultural belief in obtaining stroke care. More work is advocated among stroke survivors.

6. Strength and limitations and recommendations

The strength of this baseline study is the observation of lack of awareness and community screening, especially among stroke survivors. A study of one herbal centre is severely underpowered to draw any generalised meaningful conclusions. There is need to extend study to more survivors, and more herbal centres. One limitation here was the difficulty in having research access to most Herbal centres. The second was that majority of the herbal centres lacked proper structural organisation to allow for meaningful research work. There was also our inability to obtain body-mass index of the survivors due to lack of cooperation in this regard. This baseline study of stroke in an herbal centre should instigate more work in this area, particularly in the sub-Saharan Africa, where patronage is on the increase.

Acknowledgements

The authors wish to acknowledge the cooperation and kind support of Mr. Bebe and all staff of Bebe Herbal Centre, Umunomo, Ihitteafoukwu, Ahiazu Mbaise, Nigeria in the course of this work. We also acknowledge the contributions of Sunday Osonwa and Nkechi Chukwu in doing excellent interview work.

Sources of funding

Funds for this study were contributed from the private budget of the authors. There was no outside funding support.

Conflict of interest

The authors declare that there is no conflict of interest.

Author details

Polycarp Umunna Nwoha[1,2*], Florence Osita Okoro[2,3], Emmanuel Chukwudi Nwoha[2,4], Augustine Obi[2,5], Chidinma Oluchi Nwoha[2,6], Iyanu Ayoola[1], Nkeiru Christiana Ogoko[2], Peace Ngozi Nwoha[2,7], Anna Idaguko[2,8], Catherine Wali[2,9], Nnenna Chinagozi-Amanze[2,10] and Ifeoma H. Nwoha-Okpara[2,11]

1 Department of Anatomy and Cell Biology, Obafemi Awolowo University, Ile-Ife, Nigeria

2 Centre for Scientific Investigations and Training, Owerri, Imo State, Nigeria

3 School of Nursing, College of Health and Human Services, University of North Carolina at Charlotte, USA

4 Bucks New University, United Kingdom

5 Department of Anatomy and Neurobiology, Imo State University, Owerri, Nigeria

6 Health Centre, University of Medical Sciences, Ondo City, Ondo State, Nigeria

7 Celon Clinic, Ibeju-Lekki, Lagos State, Nigeria

8 Edo State University, Iyamho, Edo State, Nigeria

9 Baze University, Abuja, Nigeria

10 St. Catherine's Specialist Hospital Port Harcourt, Rivers State, Nigeria

11 Liviashammah Hospitals Ltd, Maraba, Nasarawa State, Nigeria

*Address all correspondence to: polycarpnwoha@yahoo.com

References

[1] Strong K, Mathers C, Bonita R. Preventing stroke: Saving lives around the world. Lancet Neurology. 2007;**6**:182-187. DOI: 10.1016/S1474-4422(07)70031-5]

[2] Lopez AD, Mathers CD, Ezzati M, Jamison DT, Murray CJ. Global and regional burden of disease and risk factors, 2001: Systematic analysis of population health data. Lancet. 2006;**367**:1747-1757. DOI: 10.1016/S0140-6736(06)687709

[3] Global Burden on Disease Collaborators 2016 reported how stroke kills per year - GBD 2016 Causes of Death Collaborators. Global, regional, and national age-sex specific mortality for 264 causes of death. 1980-2016: A systematic analysis for the global burden of disease study 2016. Lancet. 2017;**390**:1151-1210. DOI: 10.1016/S0140-6736(17)32152-9]

[4] Bravata DM, Wells CK, Gulanski B, Kernan WN, Brass LM, Long J, et al. 1997 racial disparities in stroke risk factors. Stroke. 2005;**36**:1507-1511

[5] Murray CJL, Lopez AD. Mortality by cause for eight regions of the world: Global burden of disease study. Lancet. 1997;**349**:1269

[6] Feigin VL, Krishnamurthi RV, Parmar P, Norrving B, Mensh GA, Bennett DA, et al. Update on the global burden of ischemic and hemorrhagic stroke in 1990-2013: The GBD 2013 study. Neuroepidemiology. 2015;**45**: 161-176. DOI: 10.1159/000441085]

[7] Walker R, Whiting D, Unwin N, et al. Stroke incidence in rural and urban Tanzania: A prospective, community-based study. Lancet Neurology. 2010;**7**: 786-792

[8] Owolabi MO, Akarolo-Anthony S, Akinyemi R, et al. The burden of stroke in Africa: A glance at the present and a glimpse into the future. Cardiovascular Journal of Africa. 2015;**26**(2 H3Africa Suppl):S27-S38

[9] Ejimofor MC, Uthman OA, Maduka O, et al. Stroke survivors in Nigeria: A door-to-door survey from the Niger Delta region. Journal of Neurological Sciences. 2017;**372**:262-269

[10] Akinyemi RO, Owolabi MO, Ihara M, et al. Stroke, cerebrovascular diseases and vascular cognitive improvement in Africa. Brain Research Bulletin. 2019;**145**:97-108

[11] Akinkugbe OO, Bademosi O, Osuntokun BO, et al. Incidence of stroke in an African city. Results from stroke registry at Ibadan, Nigeria 1973-1975. Stroke. 1979;**10**:205-207 It was stated that 23% of Africans run the risk of stroke in their lifetime

[12] GBD 2016 and Injury Incidence and Prevalence Collaborators. Global, regional, and national incidence, prevalence, and years lived with disability for 328 diseases and injuries for 195 countries, 1990-2016: A systematic analysis for the global burden of disease study 2016. The Lancet. 2017;**390**:1211-1259

[13] Bravata DM, Wells CL, Gulanski B, Kernan WN, Brass LM, Long J, et al. Racial disparities in stroke risk factors. Stroke. 2005;**36**:1507-1511

[14] Sacco RL, Benjamin EJ, Broderick JP, Dyken M, Easton JD, Wm F, et al. American heart association prevention conference, IV: Prevention and rehabilitation of stroke: Risk factors. Stroke. 1997;**28**:1507-1517

[15] Yang Q, Tong X, Schieb L, Vaughan A, Gillespie C, Wiltz JL, et al. Vital signs: Recent trends in stroke death rates – United States, 2000 – 2015. MMWR. Morbidity and Mortality Weekly Report. 2017;**66**:933-939. DOI: 10.15585/mmwr.mm6635e1

[16] Nwoha PU, Obi AU, Okoro FO, Waritimi GE, Ayoola IO, Eze MA, et al. Characteristics of stroke attendants at Bebe herbal center. Journal of Environment Neuroscience & Biomedicine. 2017;**4**(1):396-406

[17] Cooper RS, Amoah AGB, Mensah GA. High blood pressure: The foundation for epidemic cardiovascular disease in African populations. Ethnicity and Disease. 2003;**13**(2 Suppl. 2):S48-S52

[18] Rosenthal T, Alter A. Occupational stress and hypertension. Journal of the American Society of Hypertension. 2012;**6**(1):2-22. DOI: 10.1016/j.jash.2011.09.002

[19] Meng L, Chen D, Yang Y, Zheng Y, Hui R. Depression increases the risk of hypertension incidence: A meta-analysis of prospective cohort studies. Journal of Hypertension. 2012;**30**(5):842-851. DOI: 10.1097/HJH.0b013e32835080b7

[20] Pan Y, Cai W, Cheng Q, Dong W, An T, Yan J. Association between anxiety and hypertension: A systematic review and meta-analysis of epidemiological studies. Neuropsychiatric Disease and Treatment. 2015;**11**:1121-1130. DOI: 10.2147/NDT.S77710

[21] Everson-Rose SA, Lewis TT. Psychosocial factors and cardiovascular diseases. Annual Review of Public Health. 2005;**26**(1):469-500. DOI: 10.1146/annurev.pubhealth.26.021304.144542

[22] Spruill TM. Chronic psychosocial stress and hypertension. Current Hypertension Reports. 2010;**12**(1):10-16. DOI: 10.1007/s11906-009-0084-8

[23] Black PH, Garbutt LD. Stress, inflammation and cardiovascular disease. Journal of Psychosomatic Research. 2002;**52**(1):1-23

[24] Feigin VL, Nguyen G, et al. Global regional, and country-specific lifetime risks of stroke, 1990 and 2016. New England Journal of Medicine. 2018;**379**:2429-2437

[25] Fidelis L, Burt V, Cutler J, Hughes J, Roccella E, Sorlie P. The burden of adult hypertension in the United States; a rising tide. Hypertension. 2004;**44**:398-404

[26] Mozaffarian D, Benjamin EJ, Go AS, et al. Executive summary: Heart disease and stroke statistics – 2016 update. Circulation. 2016;**133**(4):447-454. DOI: 1161/CIR.0000000000000363

[27] Wiredu EK, Nyame PK. Stroke mortality in Accra: A study of risk factors. Ghana Medical Journal. 2001;**35**(4):151-156

[28] Nyame PK, Bonsu-Bruce N, Amoah AGB, Adjei S, Nyako E, Amuah EA, et al. Current trends in the incidence of cerebrovascular accidents in Accra. The West African Medical Journal. 1994;**3**:183-186

[29] Teppala S, Shankar A, Ducatman A. The association between acculturation and hypertension in a multiethnic sample of US adults. Journal of the American Society of Hypertension. 2010;**4**(5): 236-243. DOI: 10.1016/j.jash.2010.07.001. [Pubmed] [Google Schlar]

[30] Nwoha PU, Okoro FO, Nwoha EC, Chukwu FN, Nwoha CO, Ogoko NC, et al. Sex, knowledge and attitude of stroke survivors attending Bebe

herbal center on risk factors before and after stroke. Stroke Research and Treatment. 2021; 8 pages;**2021**:6695522. DOI: 10.1155/2021/6695522, 2021

[31] Cuffee Y, Ogedegbe C, Williams NJ, Ogedegbe G, Schnoenthaler A. Psychosocial risk factors for hypertension: An update of the literature. Current Hypertension Reports. 2014;**16**(10):483. DOI: 10.1007/s11906-0483-3

[32] Okoro FO, Nwoha CO, Ogoko NC, Nwoha EC, Amadi CC, Nwoha PN, et al. Stroke Survivors'Preference of herbal center to hospital. International Journal of Complementary Medicine. 2022;7:39. DOI: 10.28933/ijtcm-2021-11-1505

[33] World Health Organisation Regional Office for Europe, The Stroke Council. Pan European Consensus Meeting on Stroke Management: Report, Helsingber, Sweden, November 8-10, 1995. Geneva Switzerland: WHO Publications; 1996

[34] Fogelholm R, Murros K, Rissanen A, Ilmavita M. Factors delaying hospital admission after acute stroke. Stroke. 1996;**27**:398-401

[35] Onwuekwe IO, Adikaibe AE, Ohaegbulam SC, Chikani MC, Amuta J, Uloh HN. Stroke mimics – A study of CT images in Nigerian African stroke patients. Journal of Neurological Sciences (Turkish). 2008;**25**:148-154

[36] Wahab KW. The burden of stroke in Nigeria. International Journal of Stroke. 2008;**3**:290-292

[37] Bell-Gam HI, Onwuchekwa A, Iyagba A. Improving stroke management through specialized stroke units in Nigeria: A situation review. The Nigerian Health Journal. 2012;**2**:31-34

[38] Donkor ES, Owolabi MO, Bampoh P, Aspelund T, Gudnason V. Community awareness of stroke in Accra, Ghana. BMC Public Health. 2014;**14**:196

[39] Pandian JD, Sethi V, Dhillon R, Kaur R, Padala S, Chakpavorty R, et al. Is intravenous thrombolysis feasible in a developing country? Cerebrovascular Diseases. 2005;**20**:134-136

[40] Samsa GP, Cohen SJ, Goldstein LB, Bonito AJ, Duncan PW, Enarson C, et al. Knowledge of risk factors among patients at increased risk for stroke. Stroke. 1997;**28**:916-921

[41] Lionel H, Opie, Seedat YK. Hypertension in sub-Saharan Africa populations. Circulation. 2005;**112**(23): 3562-3568. DOI: 10.1161/CIRCULATION AHA. 105, 539569

Section 3

Post-Stroke Rehabilitation: Management

Chapter 5

Role of Yoga and Spirituality in Stroke Rehabilitation

Pratap Sanchetee

Abstract

In spite of the best treatment, 30–50% of stroke survivors are left with significant physical and/or psychological disabilities and consequent decline in quality of life (QOL). The silver lining is that up to 80% of stroke survivors can become independent in activities of daily living with adequate rehabilitation. Rehabilitation with physiotherapy, occupational therapy, and speech therapy offers a good opportunity to regain functional abilities. However, there is a shortage of neurorehabilitation (NR) programs across the globe, more so in resource-poor countries. The secular practice of yoga and spirituality is associated with a host of physical, physiological, cognitive, and psychological benefits that can be effectively included in stroke rehabilitation (SR). It has been shown to increase creativity and reduce stress as well as improve muscle power, dexterity, visual perception, and reaction time. These practices promote the positive effects on carotid atherosclerosis, hypertension, diabetes, and coronary artery disease, which are all identified risk factors associated with stroke occurrence or reoccurrence. Yoga and relevant practices are low cost and have good acceptance amongst patients and caregivers. In spite of yoga and meditation as useful tool, it has not been addressed adequately in stroke rehabilitation.

Keywords: yoga, spirituality, neurorehabilitation, stroke rehabilitation, neuropsychiatric complications, stress

1. Introduction

Stroke is the leading cause of disability across the globe and with better care, more people are living following stroke with mild to severe neurologic deficits. This has a negative impact on both psychological and physical health and quality of life [1]. The majority of such patients reach the plateau of their recovery within 6 months [2]. It has been observed that a good and sustainable rehabilitation program can result in improvement in muscle power, balance, mobility, risk of fall, and aerobic capacity in up to 70% of the poststroke patients [3]. Rehabilitation in stroke focuses on the recovery of function and cognition to the maximum level achievable and may include a wide range of complementary strategies including yoga [4]. The rehabilitation of stroke is a multidisciplinary process involving physicians or stroke specialists, nurses, physiotherapists, psychologists, nutritionists, occupational therapists, speech therapists, and audiologists [5, 6]. These patients require long-term rehabilitation and because of the high cost and lack of qualified therapists, they are not able to avail them. Thus, there is a strong need for novel strategies, which are low cost, suitable for home care, particularly in rural areas, and address the physical and mental needs of the patients and caregivers [7]. Yoga and meditation are such tools that are being explored in the last two decades or more. However, it is yet to find widespread acceptance. This review aims to update and synthesized the role of yoga and meditation intervention in stroke rehabilitation (SR).

2. Stroke rehabilitation

The primary purpose of rehabilitation is to maintain or improve an individual's functioning and independence. Neurorehabilitation (NR) services are essential to optimize physical, psychological, and cognitive functioning of patients with compromised neuropsychological functions especially in the initial 3–6 months poststroke [8]. There are marked inconsistencies in quality of care and rehabilitation services across the globe. Such services are needed both during the acute stage and during later phase of disease [9, 10]. NR with conventional physiotherapy, occupational therapy, and speech therapy offers them a good opportunity to regain QOL and activities of daily livings (ADLs). However, it is mostly underutilized and major barriers are limited availability, geographical distance, high cost, and lack of awareness about its benefits [8, 11, 12].

SR is a multidisciplinary process involving doctors, nurses, physiotherapists, occupational therapists, neuropsychologists, linguistic and speech specialists, audiologists, and nutritionists [13]. It is not a "one size fits all" intervention and a combination of interventions suits better to treat motor and sensory impairments, cognitive deficits, and psychological issues. Physical therapy in form of active and passive joint movement, muscle strengthening, and gait training was the cornerstone of SR till the recent past. Newer techniques such as repetitive task training (RTT), constraint-induced movement therapy (CIMT), mirror therapy, use of botulinum toxin to relieve spasticity, advanced gait training with robotic-assisted therapy and virtual reality, electrical stimulation (ES), noninvasive brain stimulation (NIBS), cognitive rehabilitation, and neurofeedback are newer addition to the armamentarium [6].

While use of technology (e.g., virtual medical examination, tele-counseling, robotic-based and exoskeleton interventions, and telerehabilitation) to manage NR has the potential to reach a large number of patients even in remote areas with limited physical contact, they have the disadvantage of complexity and high cost [8]. In this situation, yoga and spirituality as an adjunct to conventional physical and psychosocial aspects of rehabilitation merit a serious consideration [6]. Subsequent discussion in this article will focus on spirituality and yoga as an adjunct in SR.

3. Spirituality and yoga

Ancient spirituality and related practices, not synonyms with religion, are widely used for prevention of diseases, promotion of health, and as possible treatment modality for neurological and psychiatric disorders [14]. These practices include prayer, yoga, meditation, dietary modification, and mental remodeling. Recently, we are discovering their health benefits and are finding a bigger role in the field of rehabilitation [15]. They are cost-effective and self-administered options with advantages of their use in both urban and rural areas with minimal physical interactions. Spirituality and yoga, though interconnected, are different as explained below.

3.1 Spirituality

Spiritual technologies are not new to us and are guiding us through ancient times. There is no agreed definition of the term spirituality. It is a blend of humanistic psychology with an individual relationship with higher powers and the subjective experience of the "deepest values and meanings by which people live" [16–18].

To have wider application, it is necessary to distinguish spirituality from religion. While spirituality refers to a quest in life or a transcendent relationship with a higher power, religion focuses on community-based doctrine, prescribed beliefs, practices, and rituals [6, 17, 18]. Spirituality is generally considered to be a much broader construct than religious faith, although the two concepts may overlap [19]. It must be clarified that being spiritual does not necessarily mean religious, whereas the reverse is true.

As such studies relating to spirituality and rehabilitation for neurological illnesses are limited, much research is needed to evaluate their specific role [1, 17]. Though higher levels of spirituality are known to be associated with a better quality of life (QOL) for people with neurodisability and their caregivers, most of the medical staff are not well equipped to administer it [20, 21].

3.2 Yoga and meditation

Yoga is a way of life and an ancient mind-body practice that originated in India more than 5,000 years ago. It is now recognized worldwide to have spiritual, physical, and mental health benefits [1, 22, 23]. The word "yoga" is derived from Sanskrit verb "*yuj*" meaning to yoke or unite. Commonly, yoga is translated to imply the union of body, mind, and spirit [22, 24]. Meditation in its many forms has been practiced over millions of years by diverse groups of people in many different traditions. In a more modern context, it can be defined as "a systematic practice and implementation of mind and body in the living process of human beings to keep harmony within self, within society, and with nature" [25].

There are many practices of yoga and they include varying combinations of spiritual way of life, different bodily postures (*asanas*), controlled breathing (*pranayam*), physical and mental relaxation, contemplation, control of thoughts and mind (concentration meditation), and open-mindedness or mindfulness [1, 14, 22]. Meditation, the most important component of yoga, aims at giving peace to the mind and increasing awareness of environment and higher consciousness.

The practices of yoga and meditation strengthen willpower and control of mind and body to work in perfect synergy [1, 13]. They are known to promote cardio-respiratory and metabolic health (reduction of carotid atherosclerosis, dyslipidemia, hypertension, diabetes, and coronary artery disease) and as a possible treatment modality for a variety of neurological and psychosomatic disorders [1, 22, 26].

4. Mechanism of improvement in stroke with yoga

Though yoga and spiritual techniques-based practices are becoming increasingly popular in the management of many physical and psychological illnesses, the neurobiological effects of such practices in improvement are not well understood [4, 27, 28]. It must be appreciated that unlike majority of conventional SR techniques aims at deficit recovery (external mechanism), spirituality and yoga work at intrinsic recovery of the brain as well. Neuropsychological studies have shown that mindfulness meditation training improves immunity, cognitive skills (thinking, reasoning, judgment, and memory), attention-related behavioral responses and emotional liability, and reduction in autonomic arousal [1, 27].

4.1 Autonomic nervous system

There is increasing support for the theory that relates the positive effects of yoga to a close link between the central nervous system and the autonomic nervous system, along with the endocrine and immune systems. It is believed that yoga techniques favor a down-regulation of the hypothalamic-pituitary-adrenal (HPA) axis and the sympathetic nervous system (SNS), leading to a prevalence of the parasympathetic nervous system over the SNS, possibly through direct vagal stimulation [4]. Moreover, breathing control and meditation practices in yoga increase the autonomic control, and reduce blood pressure, heart rate, and breathing. These changes may help in poststroke rehabilitation through restoration of physical and mental health, promotion and coordination of complex movements, balance, strengthening, and breathing.

4.2 Hormonal changes

The stress hormones (such as cortisol) that compromise the immune system can be balanced through practice of yoga [29]. The practice of yoga enhances the activity of many hormones connected with mental health such as melatonin and gamma aminobutyric acid (GABA) [30, 31].

There are pieces of evidence that meditation-based training increases many growth factors such as brain-derived neurotrophic factor (BDNF), nerve growth factor (NGF), vascular endothelial growth factor (VEGF), hepatocyte growth factor (HGF), glial-derived thrombospondin 1 and 2, and growth-inducing proteins (neuromodulin, CAP23, MARCKS) [32]. Higher levels of these growth factors are associated with better neuroplasticity, neuronal morphology (synaptic and dendritic changes), and cortical reorganization improving functional outcomes following neurological illnesses.

4.3 Brain structures

Till recently, it was believed neural tissues do not regenerate. Now, we have learned that it is possible to reconstruct neural circuits with transplanted endogenous neural stem cells or through mental training such as meditation [33, 34]. Long practice with yoga has been associated with changing brain structures with an increase in gray matter density in structures involving memory, attention, self-awareness, compassion, and control of the autonomic nervous system [27, 33]. Functional magnetic resonance imaging (fMRI) studies have shown increased gray matter in the hippocampus, prefrontal cortex, cingulate cortex, and brain networks including the default mode network (DMN) [1, 26, 27, 35]. In contrast to this, there was a decrease in the grey matter in the amygdala, the part of the brain associated with fear and stress.

4.4 Epigenetic

Epigenetic refers to a way to regulate gene activity in real time without modifying the DNA sequence. It allows the body to function in changing environment. Yoga and related practices have been shown to alter gene expression, particularly those related to free radical handling, inflammation processes, mitochondrial energy production and utilization, and apoptosis [1, 36, 37].

4.5 Cellular oxygenation and general well being

As a result of practice of *asanas* (body posture), *pranayam* (control of breathing), and control of thoughts and mind, there is general improvement in well-being and a positive outlook in life. With respiratory practice (*pranayam*), there is improvement in the lung capacity and respiratory health, which in turn improves supply of the oxygenated blood to multiple organs for smooth optimal function [30].

4.6 Dietary modifications

Lifestyle diseases such as obesity, accelerated atherosclerosis, insulin resistance, type 2 diabetes, and cardiovascular disease are major risk factor contributors to occurrence of stroke [38]. They are targets in both primary and secondary preventions of the stroke. Current dietary practice is loaded with a high proportion of refined carbohydrates and saturated fats. Thus, it is logical to build body-mind through diet, exercise, healthy lifestyle choices, and mental remodeling with spirituality. Spirituality and meditation techniques mandate a vegetarian diet rich in fiber content and unsaturated fats with less refined carbohydrates (**Table 1**).

• Restructuring dietary intake and fasting
• Be vegetarian and avoid nonvegetarian meals
• Plenty of fluids
• Avoid junk food
• Avoid night meals and follow intermittent fasting (with a feeding and fasting schedule of 8:16 hours)
• Adequate intake of proteins, vitamins, minerals

Table 1.
Some simple dietary principles with spiritual technologies.

5. Yoga and spirituality for stroke rehabilitation

Spirituality, meditation, and mind-body exercises are novel therapeutic approaches in improving neurological outcomes and enhancing cognitive capabilities [13, 39, 40]. Such practices allow SR in less complex and highly individualized environment. However, yoga and meditation programs should be tailored to deliver personalized interventions according to each person's profile and rehabilitation needs. Being a low cost model, it improves availability of rehabilitation in low- to middle-income countries. Though it is effective and less labor intensive, there is a lack of evidence-based review to support the claim.

Few specific practices of meditation that have been used for stroke rehabilitation are *Preksha* Meditation (based on perception theory), Qigong (Chinese body-mind exercise), and yoga-based *asanas* or exercises [11, 19, 39, 24, 32, 41–45]. A recent systematic review concluded that yoga can be used as self-administered practice in stroke rehabilitation, due to its effect on relieving the mind and body from stress. Yoga was found to act at both psychological and physical levels, and improvements were noted in self-efficacy and confidence [1, 4].

5.1 Motor and sensory functions

Rehabilitation in ICU & During acute phase: Patients with moderate-to-severe stroke are often subjected to prolonged bed rest and mechanical ventilation [13]. Such patients have a significant deficit of motor functions in form of profound muscle weakness, fatigue, diffuse myalgia, balance deficits, fear of falling (FoF), dysautonomia, orthostatic hypotension, respiratory muscle weakness, deep vein thrombosis, decubitus ulcer, joint contracture, and impaired ADLs. Neuromotor rehabilitation is a key concept of recovery from immobilization syndrome. Modified yoga (a combination of postures, breathing, and meditation) has been shown to improve vital capacity, muscle power, range of movements, walking capacity and speed, self-efficacy, and improved quality of life [11, 22, 41, 43, 46].

Rehabilitation during subacute and chronic phase: Several investigators have found improvements in muscle force, balance, aerobic capacity, timed mobility, and aphasia in subjects with chronic poststroke hemiparesis following yogic interventions [24, 39, 42]. Bastille and Gill-Body [41] demonstrated that yoga results in significant improvement in muscle power and range of movements in hemiplegic limbs and some positive effects on the Berg Balance Scale (BBS), Timed Movement Battery (TMB), and quality of life (QOL) as assessed with Stroke Impact Scale (SIS). Schmid et al. [11] in a study of 37 poststroke patients managed with yoga interventions observed significant improvement in balance (Berg Balance Scale, 41.3±11.7 vs. 46.3±9.1; $P<0.001$) and fear of fall (51% vs. 46%; $P < 0.001$). In a study carried out by Singh et al. [43], *Preksha* Meditation training was given to 22 subjects with hemiplegia and was compared with an equal number of controls at 3 months. A significant improvement was observed in muscle power and range of movements in hemiplegic limbs. In another prospective trial, Qigong practice for 16 weeks in stroke subjects was associated with improvement in balance capacity, physical well-being, and psychological well-being [44]. Psychological improvement with reduction in anxiety and depression and better QOL are additional advantages of mediation, which is helpful for patients and their caregivers [21–23, 42, 47]. Wang et al. [45] in a systemic analysis of 33 rt-fMRI neurofeedback studies on 651 healthy individuals and 15 stroke patients observed a learned modulation of brain signals, with associated changes at both the neural and the behavioral levels with this intervention.

Thus, meditation and mind-body exercises are a novel therapeutic approaches to enhance cognitive capabilities and are effective in improving poststroke outcomes [11, 21, 22, 26, 39, 40].

5.2 Cognitive rehabilitation

A large number of patients with stroke suffer from cognitive impairment. There are many types of cognitive deficits in these patients, which include forgetfulness, confusion, disorientation, problems with attention, executive functioning, information processing, etc. [48, 49]. However, cognitive rehabilitation is still far from satisfaction. Meditation and other mind-body interventions are effective in improving cognitive functions in these patients [50, 51]. However, only a small number of stroke patients have been evaluated with yoga-based interventions and Mindfulness-Based Stress Reduction (MBSR) programs in subjects with cognitive impairment. There is a requirement to study a larger number of patients and to design modified yoga program to suit different characteristics of stroke patients.

5.3 Stress and psychological

Apart from motor deficits, stroke patients have a significant cognitive deficit, stress, negative emotions, frustration, boredom, disturbed sleep, anxiety, losing a job, financial problems, depression, and behavior-related problems that hamper their recovery [8, 52]. These emotional stress results not only in *de novo* illnesses but can exacerbate preexisting illnesses as well. Some simple tips are given in **Table 2** and the list can be expanded with personal experience.

It is pertinent for us to identify stressors early and manage them accordingly. Few simple steps are
• Be friends with all livings beings
• Prefer positivity over negativity
• Gratitude to those who help
• Strengthen emotional bonding
• Watch & learn from kids & nature
• Be environment friendly
• Be happy in small acts
• Good sleep

Table 2.
Simple mental remodeling steps.

Spiritual techniques and yoga provide a good non-pharmacological approach to handling such psychological issues that are common among patients and caregivers [1, 22, 25, 49, 53]. Yoga has been demonstrated to provide relief from stressful psychological states with a reduction in anxiety, depression, and cortisol levels. Immink et al. [42] observed significant improvements in quality of life associated with a perceived motor function ($P = .0001$), perceived recovery ($P = .072$), and memory-related quality of life scores ($P = .022$), with decreases in state and trait anxiety following yoga intervention. In a recent cross-sectional, online survey of clinicians ($n > 600$) regarding coping strategies employed by them to mitigate stress was physical activity/exercise (59%), psychotherapy (26%), yoga (25%), religious or spiritual practices (23%), meditation (23%), and virtual support groups (16%) [54].

5.4 Caregivers

Developing a caregiver-driven stroke rehabilitation program has been attractive in India to address the scarcity of rehabilitation centers and trained therapists. The physical and mental health of caregivers is an important consideration in long-term SR. Spirituality and resilience needs of caregivers must be strengthened so that they can cope with the burden [8, 19].

6. Modification of yoga practices for stroke rehabilitation

While motor deficit and spasticity management in SR are well organized, the mental health program is not standardized and there is a requirement to develop a holistic module considering all aspects of rehabilitation. Spirituality and yoga are cost-effective self-administered options for SR and should find a place in the SR schedule [1, 6]. It is recommended that these interventions should be tailored to deliver personalized interventions according to each person's profile and rehabilitation needs (duration of illness and level of impairment, function and mobility, etc.).

Step description	Duration
1. Place, position, and prayer (decided on patient's condition and disablement) • Select a quiet place with least distraction. • Comfortably sitting on a chair or lying in the bed. • Prayer: Content is left to person's belief and faith. It will be either a silent one by the self or play a recorded one.	5 minutes
2. Posture (*asanas*) and loosening movements: • Based on patient's condition movements can be active, passive, or assisted. • Based on physical disablement, one can increase it to 10–15 minutes	10–15 minutes
3. *Pranayam* (breathing exercises) and controlled breathing: • Make breathing slow, long and rhythmic. Take a deep breath in with your mouth closed and hold it comfortably for 2–4 seconds. Then exhale effortlessly with mouth closed. Repeat this initially for 5 times in 2 minutes and with practice gradually increased it to 9–11 times in 7–10 min. • *Pranayam* has shown to enhance body oxygen utilization, improve concentration, and clean the respiratory passages.	7–10 minutes
4. Body relaxation with awareness (*Kayotsarga*) • Instruct body to relax each part, one by one, from the toe to the upper part of the head. Autosuggest for relaxation of muscles, body, and mind. Maintain this relaxation of body and mind initially for five minutes and with practice increase it to ten minutes.	10 minutes
5. Concentration meditation • With eyes closed focus your attention on a single object, idea, sensation, or aspect of divinity (e.g., counting or monitoring breathing, reciting a mantra, visualizing processes in the body, external object, etc.) at the exclusion of all other thoughts. Distracting thoughts will invariably appear but try to ignore them by focusing the mind through autosuggestions.	7–10 minutes
6. Open mindedness • This is a higher stage of meditation, which can be practiced after one has mastered concentration meditation. Instead of focusing attention, there is expansion of awareness and attention. All sensory inputs, be it internal (thoughts, feelings, memory, etc.) or be it external (sound, smell, etc.), are perceived as they are without any prejudice and in a nonreactive way. This provides a stimulus to gain access to knowledge, self-realization, and soul (consciousness) purification.	7–10 minutes
7. Conclusion • Gently close your meditation session with producing mahapran dhavani on two occasions. Rub your hands and move your body freely.	One minute

Table 3.
Stroke rehabilitation module with spiritual and yoga practices (To be under guidance of a physician & trained yoga teacher).

Some of the *asanas* suggested are downward-facing dog, tree pose, and child pose, and these can restore balance and significantly reduce the risk of falling for stroke patients. In view of physical limitations, practice of *asanas* should have provision for adequate support such as practice against the wall, use of head gears, etc. A suggested module as designed by the author is given in **Table 3** and should be modified as per patient's need.

7. Future

There is a good potential for spiritual technologies to be included in the NR schedule. Some of the areas that need to be considered for research are as follows:

1. Research-based modification of yoga and meditation schedule to suit disabilities, limitations, and co-morbid conditions.

2. To quantify benefits and acceptability of these technologies in a large number of people.

3. To elucidate neurobiological mechanism of these technologies in bringing the improvement.

4. To develop and amalgamate delivery of these procedures with use of low-cost technologies such as smartphones or tablets for tele-counseling, tele-training, tele-monitoring, and tele-rehabilitation.

5. To develop guidelines for use of spiritual technologies and yoga in SR.

8. Conclusions

The field of stroke rehabilitation has a bright future. In spite of good potential for recovery, these rehabilitative measures are underutilized and major barriers are limited availability, geographical distance, high cost, and lack of awareness about its benefits. Scientific evidence indicates that yoga may constitute a promising add-on therapy for a number of diseases. It is a simple to learn, adaptable and community-based practice, which could be cost-effective [1, 4]. Studies relating to spirituality and rehabilitation for neurodisability including stroke are limited [16, 17]. They can be employed at a hospital, home, and workplaces alike. Recent experiments have proved its benefit in achieving physical, mental, and spiritual health. Medical and paramedical practitioners involved in SR should be aware of them and educate the patients and caregivers.

Meditation is a body-mind exercise that could be a cost-effective and useful technique for poststroke rehabilitation [21, 23]. Though spiritual techniques are effective and less labor intensive, there is a lack of evidence-based review to support the claim. Such interventions should be considering variables such as duration of illness, type and level of impairment, and functional need. However, large-scale methodologically robust trials are required to study mobility, balance, postural stability, coordination, cognitive changes, and QOL [4]. It is recommended that yoga and meditation interventions should be designed to meet patients' different characteristics (time after stroke, level of impairment, function, and mobility). To maintain the continuum for stroke care and reduce morbidity and mortality with stroke, there is a need for public health systems in both developed and developing countries to improve stroke awareness and to implement proper strategies of triage, acute treatment, well-defined rehabilitation plans, and teleservices [8].

Funding

Nil.

Author contributions

This review was prepared by the sole author (PS).

Conflict of interest

The authors declare that the research was conducted in the absence of any commercial or financial relationships that could be construed as a potential conflict of interest.

Abbreviation

QOL	Quality of life
NR	Neurorehabilitation
SR	Stroke rehabilitation

Author details

Pratap Sanchetee
Sanchetee Neurology Research Institute, Jodhpur, Rajasthan, India

*Address all correspondence to: pratap.sanchetee@gmail.com

References

[1] Lazaridou A, Philbrook P, Tzika AA. Yoga and mindfulness as therapeutic interventions for stroke rehabilitation: A systematic review. Evidence Based Complementary Alternative Medicine. 2013;**76**:9

[2] Jørgensen HS, Nakayama H, Raaschou HO, Vive-Larsen J, Støier M, Olsen TS. Outcome and time course of recovery in stroke. Part II: Time course of recovery. The Copenhagen Stroke Study. Archives of Physical Medicine and Rehabilitation. 1995;**76**(5):406-412. DOI: 10.1016/s0003-9993(95)80568-0

[3] Weiss A, Suzuki T, Bean J, Fielding RA. High intensity strength training improves strength and functional performance after stroke. American Journal of Physical Medicine & Rehabilitation. 2000;**79**(4):369-376

[4] Lawrence M, Celestino Junior FT, Matozinho HH, Govan L, Booth J, Beecher J. Yoga for stroke rehabilitation. Cochrane Database System Review. 2017;**12**(12):CD011483

[5] Alessandro L, Olmos LE, Bonamico L, et al. Rehabilitación multidisciplinaria para pacientes adultos con accidente cerebrovascular [Multidisciplinary rehabilitation for adult patients with stroke]. Medicina (B Aires). 2020;**80**(1):54-68

[6] Sanchetee P. Ischemic Stroke. London: IntechOpen; 2022

[7] Sheehy LM. Considerations for postacute rehabilitation for survivors of COVID-19. JMIR Public Health and Surveillance. 2020;**6**(2):e19462. DOI: 10.2196/19462

[8] Sylaja PN, Srivastava MVP, Shah S, Bhatia R, Khurana D, Sharma A, et al. The SARS-CoV-2/COVID-19 pandemic and challenges in stroke care in India. Annals of New York Academy Science. 2020;**1473**:3-10

[9] Bryant SE, McNabb K. Postintensive care syndrome. Critical Care Nursing Clinics of North America. 2019;**31**:507-516. DOI: 10.1016/j.cnc.2019.07.006

[10] Garg RK. Spectrum of neurological manifestations in Covid-19: A review. Neurology India. 2020;**68**:560-572. DOI: 10.4103/0028-3886.289000

[11] Schmid AA, Van Puymbroeck M, Altenburger PA, Schalk NL, Dierks TA, Miller KK, et al. Poststroke balance improves with yoga: A pilot study. Stroke. 2012;**43**:2402-2407

[12] Smith MA, Tomita MR. Combined effects of telehealth and modified constraint-induced movement therapy for individuals with chronic hemiparesis. International Journal of Telerehabilitation. 2020;**12**(1):51-62. DOI: 10.5195/ijt.2020.6300

[13] Brugliera L, Spina A, Castellazzi P, Cimino P, Tettamanti A, Houdayer E, et al. Rehabilitation of COVID-19 patients. Journal of Rehabilitation Medicine. 2020;**52**(4):jrm00046

[14] Mishra SK, Singh P, Bunch SJ, Zhang R. The therapeutic value of yoga in neurological disorders. Annals of Indian Academy of Neurology. 2012;**15**(4):247-254. DOI: 10.4103/0972-2327.104328

[15] Alanagreh L, Alzoughool F, Atoum M. The human coronavirus disease COVID-19: Its origin, characteristics, and insights into potential drugs and its mechanisms.

Pathogens. 2020;**9**(5):331. DOI: 10.3390/pathogens9050331

[16] Miller WR, Thoresen CE. Spirituality, religion, and health: An emerging research field. The American Psychologist. 2003;**58**(1):24-35

[17] Dein S. Religion, spirituality and neurorehabilitation. NeuroRehabilitation. 2020;**46**(1):1-2. DOI: 10.3233/NRE-200001

[18] Wikipedia. Spirituality. Available from: https://en.wikipedia.org/wiki/Spirituality. [Accessed: 24 May 2022]

[19] Gibbs LAL, Anderson MI, Simpson GK, Jones KF. Spirituality and resilience among family caregivers of survivors of stroke: A scoping review. NeuroRehabilitation. 2020;**46**(1):41-52. DOI: 10.3233/NRE-192946

[20] Fionaa JK, Juliea P, Candicea CU, Kenneth SG. Rehabilitation health professionals' perceptions of spirituality and spiritual care: The results of an online survey. NeuroRehabilitation. 2020;**46**(1):17-30. DOI: 10.3233/NRE-192857

[21] Pucciarelli G, Vellone E, Bolgeo T, Simeone S, Alvaro R, Lee CS, et al. Role of spirituality on the association between depression and quality of life in stroke survivor-care partner dyads. Circulation. Cardiovascular Quality and Outcomes. 2020;**13**(6):e006129. DOI: 10.1161/CIRCOUTCOMES.119.006129

[22] Sanchetee P, Jain A, Agarwal H. Preksha meditation and mental health in elderly. Journal of Indian Academy Geriatrics. 2017;**13**(7):131

[23] Falkenberg RI, Eising C, Peters ML. Yoga and immune system functioning: A systematic review of randomized controlled trials. Journal of Behavioral Medicine. 2018;**41**:467-482

[24] Paldhikar S, Kulkarni G, Ghodey S, Sutar A. Effects of yoga-based exercises on balance in chronic post-stroke patients. International Journal of Physiotherapy Research. 2016;**4**:1766

[25] Sharma M. Yoga as an alternative and complementary approach for stress management: A systematic review. J Evidence-Based Complementary & Alternative Medicine. 2014;**19**(1):59-67

[26] Telles S, Naveen KV. Yoga for rehabilitation: An overview. Indian Journal of Medical Sciences. 1997;**51**:123-127

[27] Mayo KR. Support from neurobiology for spiritual techniques for anxiety: A brief review. Journal of Health Care Chaplaincy. 2010;**16**:53-57

[28] Pascoe MC, Thompson DR, Ski CF. Yoga, mindfulness-based stress reduction and stress-related physiological measures: A meta-analysis. Psychoneuroendocrinology. 2017;**86**:152-168. DOI: 10.1016/j.psyneuen.2017.08.008

[29] Mahajan AS. Role of yoga in hormonal homeostasis. International Journal of Clinical Experimental Physiology. 2014;**1**(3):173-178

[30] Bernardi L, Spadacini G, Bellwon J, Hajric R, Roskamm H, Frey AW. Effect of breathing rate on oxygen saturation and exercise performance in chronic heart failure. The Lancet. 2016;**351**(9112):1308-1311. DOI: 10.1016/S0140-6736(97)10341-5

[31] Bushell W, Castle R, Williams MA, Brouwer KC, Tanzi RE, Chopra D, et al. Meditation and yoga practices as potential adjunctive treatment of

SARS-CoV-2 infection and COVID-19: A brief overview of key subjects. Journal of Alternative and Complementary Medicine. 2020;**26**(7):547-556. DOI: 10.1089/acm.2020.0177

[32] Okazaki H, Beppu H, Mizutani K, Okamoto S, Sonoda S. Changes in serum growth factors in stroke rehabilitation patients and their relation to hemiparesis improvement. Journal of Stroke and Cerebrovascular Diseases. 2014;**23**(6):1703-1708. DOI: 10.1016/j.jstrokecerebrovasdis.2014.01.015

[33] Lazar SW, Kerr CE, Wasserman RH, Gray JR, Greve DN, Treadway MT, et al. Meditation experience is associated with increased cortical thickness. Neuroreport. 2005;**16**(17):1893-1897. DOI: 10.1097/01.wnr.0000186598.66243.19

[34] Ito A, Kubo N, Liang N, Aoyama T, Kuroki H. Regenerative rehabilitation for stroke recovery by inducing synergistic effects of cell therapy and neurorehabilitation on motor function: A narrative review of pre-clinical studies. International Journal of Molecular Science. 2020;**21**(9):3135

[35] Gothe NP, Khan I, Hayes J, Erlenbach E, Damoiseauxb JS. Yoga effects on brain health: A systematic review of the current literature. Brain Plast. 2019;**5**(1):105-122

[36] Bhasin MK, Dusek JA, Chang BH, et al. Relaxation response induces temporal transcriptome changes in energy metabolism, insulin secretion and inflammatory pathways. PLoS One. 2013;**8**(5):e62817

[37] Venditti S, Verdone L, Reale A, Vetriani V, Caserta M, Zampieri M. Molecules of silence: Effects of meditation on gene expression and epigenetics. Frontiers in Psychology. 2020;**11**:1767. DOI: 10.3389/fpsyg.2020.01767

[38] Demasi M. COVID-19 and metabolic syndrome: Could diet be the key? BMJ Evidence Based Medicine. 2021;**26**(1):1-2. DOI: 10.1136/bmjebm-2020-111451

[39] Lynton H, Kligler B, Shiflett S. Yoga in stroke rehabilitation: A systematic review and results of a pilot study. Topics in Stroke Rehabilitation. 2007;**14**(4):1-8. DOI: 10.1310/tsr1404-1

[40] Silveira K, Smart CM. Cognitive, physical, and psychological benefits of yoga for acquired brain injuries: A systematic review of recent findings. Neuropsychological Rehabilitation. 2020;**30**(7):1388-1407. DOI: 10.1080/09602011.2019.1583114

[41] Bastille JV, Gill-Body KM. A Yoga-based exercise program for people with chronic poststroke hemiparesis. Physical Therapy. 2004;**84**:33-48

[42] Immink MA, Hillier S, Petkov J. Randomized controlled trial of yoga for chronic poststroke hemiparesis: Motor function, mental health, and quality of life outcomes. Topics in Stroke Rehabilitation. 2014;**21**(3):256-271. DOI: 10.1310/tsr2103-256

[43] Singh PS, Singh A, Mishra JPN. Management of hemiplegia through Preksha meditation. International Journal of Yoga Allied Science. 2014;**3**(2):143-149

[44] Yuen MSM, Lau PMY, Chau RMW, Chen TMK, Pang MYC. Qigong could be an effective and alternative complementary management for post-stroke rehabilitation: Preliminary results. Cerebrovasular Diseases. 2017;**44**:50

[45] Wang T, Mantini D, Gillebert CR. The potential of real-time fMRI neurofeedback for stroke rehabilitation: A systematic review. Cortex. 2018;**107**:148-165. DOI: 10.1016/j.cortex.2017.09.006

[46] Streeter CC, Gerbarg PL, Saper RB, Ciraulo DA, Brown RP. Effects of yoga on the autonomic nervous system, gamma-aminobutyric-acid, and allostasis in epilepsy, depression, and post-traumatic stress disorder. Medical Hypotheses. 2012;**78**(5):571-579. DOI: 10.1016/j.mehy.2012.01.021

[47] Kabat-Zinn J, Lipworth L, Burney R. The clinical use of mindfulness meditation for the self-regulation of chronic pain. Journal of Behavioral Medicine. 1985;**8**(2):163-190

[48] Zarrabian S, Hassani-Abharian P. COVID-19 Pandemic and the importance of cognitive rehabilitation. Basic Clinical Neuroscience. 2020;**11**(2):129-132

[49] Froeliger B, Garland EL, Mclernon FJ. Yoga meditation practitioners exhibit greater gray matter volume and fewer reported cognitive failures: Results of a preliminary voxel-based morphometric analysis. Evidence-Based Complementary and Alternative Medicine. 2012;**2012**:821307

[50] Jedrczak A, Toomey M, Clements G. The TM-Sidhi program, age and brief tests of perceptual-motor speed and nonverbal intelligence. Journal of Clinical Psychology. 1986;**42**(1):161-164

[51] Brunner D, Abramovitch A, Etherton J. A yoga program for cognitive enhancement. PLoS One. 2017;**12**(8):e0182366

[52] Nagarathna R, Nagendra HR, Majumdar V. A perspective on yoga as a preventive strategy for coronavirus disease. International Journal of Yoga. 2020;**13**(2):89-98. DOI: 10.4103/ijoy.IJOY_22_20

[53] Francis AL, Beemer RC. How does yoga reduce stress? Embodied cognition and emotion highlight the influence of the musculoskeletal system. Complementary Therapies in Medicine. 2019;**43**:170-175

[54] Shechter A, Diaz F, Moise N, Anstey DE, Ye S, Agarwal S, et al. Psychological distress, coping behaviors, and preferences for support among New York healthcare workers during the COVID-19 pandemic. General Hospital Psychiatry. 2020;**66**:1-8

Chapter 6

Microbiome-Based Interventions: A New Prospect in Post-Stroke Rehabilitation

Mubarak Muhammad, Rabi'u Musa Isah and Abdurrazak Muhammad

Abstract

Post-stroke rehabilitation remains the preferred therapeutic option for stroke survivors due to its unrestrictive therapeutic window of unlimited lifelong applicability. However, post-stroke rehabilitative interventions are still far from ideal and optimal recovery from lost functions after stroke. This heralds the search for strategies to complement rehabilitative interventions. Expanding the armamentarium of the existing post-stroke rehabilitation strategies will go a long way towards the attainment of optimal functions lost due to stroke. One of the promising emerging trends in stroke is cherished within the microbiome present in the gastrointestinal system. There is bidirectional communication between stroke and gut microbiome via gut-brain axis, and plethora of evidence pointed that modulation of this axis impact on stroke outcome, as well as evidence linking gut microbiome in modulation of brain neuroplasticity. Herein, we explored evidence that will support future research and perspectives into the potentiality of microbiome-based interventions as an integral part of post-stroke rehabilitation. Findings support the premise of the function of gut microbiome in brain neuroplasticity, and this could be fundamental towards translating similar phenomenon in human stroke to promote brain neuroplasticity in complement with post-stroke rehabilitation.

Keywords: microbiome, microbiota, microbiota gut-brain axis, stroke, post-stroke rehabilitation, neuroplasticity

1. Introduction

A stroke occurs due to interruptions in blood supply to the brain, and over the years stroke consistently constitutes the second most common cause of mortality after cardiovascular diseases and a foremost root of chronic adult disability [1–3]. Individuals that survive stroke experience a multifaceted range of impairments as a result of loss of brain function due to the infarct, with acute clinical treatment of those impairments tailored towards rescuing the larger component of potentially affected but yet viable neurons in the ischemic penumbra that surround the ischemic core [4]. However, the approved strategy to salvage neurons in the ischemic penumbra using recombinant tissue plasminogen activator (rtPA) and mechanical thrombectomy remains largely unsatisfactory and is only available to an only small fraction of about 5% of stroke patients due to narrow time of applicability within 4.5 h of stroke onset [5]. Moreover, despite advancement in understanding the mechanism of neuronal demise after stroke and the corresponding development of neuroprotective agents, translating findings from bench to bedside has been largely disappointing, as about 70 agents tested in more than 140 clinical trials have all been unsatisfying [6].

Therefore, post-stroke rehabilitation aims at restoring functional impairments as well as promoting better compensation of the resulting defects after stroke remains a favorite therapeutic option against stroke due to its relative advantage of unrestrictive time of applicability [7]. Rehabilitative interventions are principally based on modifying and boosting the neuronal plasticity processes [8, 9]. Neuroplasticity is a general term used to denote the life-long natural capability of the nervous system to act in response to intrinsic or extrinsic stimuli by rearranging itself in terms of structural, functional, and molecular form [10]. There are numerous processes of neuroplasticity that allow for neuronal reorganization, which includes neurogenesis, gliogenesis, angiogenesis, synaptogenesis, dendritic arborization, axonal sprouting, long-term potentiation (LTP), enrollment of other pathways, strengthening of functionally silent synapses. Thus, the categorization into neuronal plasticity (neurogenesis), synaptic plasticity (LTP), and global plasticity is often used to take into account the various organizational level of neuroplasticity. Brain injury, due to stroke, is one of the potent stimuli that lead to the activation of neuroplasticity processes to initiate spontaneous recovery. The rehabilitative interventions take advantage of this endogenous brain capacity to promote it as well as remodel it in the right direction to achieve maximum recovery from functional impairment after stroke [11, 12].

Nevertheless, it was estimated that about 50% of individuals that survived stroke are left with residual functional impairment even with rehabilitative interventions [13]. This prompted the search for strategies that enhance neuroplasticity to complement rehabilitative interventions. Various strategies to achieve that using transcranial direct current stimulation, functional electrical stimulation, deep brain stimulation, brain-derived neurotrophic factor (BDNF) therapy, Statins therapy, erythropoietin (EPO) therapy, phosphodiesterase type 5 inhibitors, and vascular endothelial growth factor (VEGF) therapy have all been under investigation [4]. But considerations for gut microbiome-based interventions to enhance neuroplasticity and supplement neuro-rehabilitation of stroke have not been explored. This is despite the fact that there exists numerous evidence indicating mechanistic link implicating gut microbiome in the pathogenesis of stroke and mediating through gut microbiome to impact on stroke outcome [14–17], as well the role microbiome as a potential modulator of brain neuroplasticity [18].

Gut microbiome is composed of a complex community of trillions of microbes, consisting of bacteria, fungi, viruses, archaea, and protozoa, with bacteria constituting more than 90% of the gastrointestinal ecosystem [19–22]. The mechanism through which the gut microbiome mediates an integral role in the pathogenesis of stroke has been well established [23]. Brain lesion due to stroke together with the effect from stroke-induced immunosuppression caused harmful consequences on gut microbiome via top-down signaling of microbiota gut-brain axis. Such consequences include dysbiosis, imbalance in resident intestinal immune function, and intestinal barrier dysfunction [24]. The bottom-up signaling of microbiota gut-brain axis through microbiome associated effect in up-regulation in pro-inflammatory immune cells and cytokines, as well as an increase in permeability of microbes and their components, lead to compounding effect on stroke injury by escalating neuro-inflammation and unsettling in integrity of blood–brain barrier (BBB) [25]. In this paper, therefore, we explored evidence that will support future research and perspectives into the potentiality of microbiome-based interventions as an integral part of post-stroke rehabilitation.

2. Post-stroke rehabilitation and neuroplasticity

Post-stroke rehabilitation entails healthcare that manages post-stroke disability and the underline condition that cause or accompany the stroke, with the goal that focuses on reducing the disability and enhancing the performance in activities of daily living (ADL). Because post-stroke rehabilitation objectives are complex and dynamic involving measures to avoid further decline in function, optimize the existing function, and reach for the highest possible level of independence (physically, psychologically, socially, and financially) possible, multidisciplinary interventions from a number of disciplines are employed [26]. Post-stroke rehabilitation guidelines are therefore developed based on evidence-based best data to improve and support the best clinical rehabilitation of stroke [27, 28]. Nevertheless, even with the best clinical practice in post-stroke rehabilitation, certain populations of stroke survivors are still living with residual disabilities. Rehabilitation as a process generally explores the basis for brain recovery from impairments, which are adaptation, restitution, and neuroplasticity [29].

Recovery in function in post-stroke brain depends majorly on neuroplasticity. Neuroplasticity entails the inherent capability of the CNS to change structurally and functionally as a result of new experiences [30]. There exist many techniques to detect neuroplasticity in the human brain. The most frequently used include functional magnetic resonance imaging (fMRI) which assesses changes in activation and recruitment of brain regions and noninvasive brain stimulation which can detect a change in volume, location, and excitability of motor cortical maps [31]. The basic processes in learning-related plasticity include the amplification of existing neuronal connections, as well as the formation of new connections to support learned behaviors [32]. These processes are then followed by synaptic pruning of the connections as skill and preferential pathways develop. For this, one of the current approaches to optimize the functional benefits of post-stroke motor rehabilitation is by focusing on interventions that encourage motor learning-related neuroplasticity [31].

The molecular level of synaptic plasticity has been extensively studied. In synaptic plasticity, there is exocytosis of neurotransmitters to modulate synaptic plasticity either at monosynaptic or multi-synaptic level, thus neurotransmitter-receptor binding is critical to synaptic plasticity [33]. Within the cortex, glutamate receptors play a key role, as glutamate is the most important excitatory neurotransmitter. The arrival of impulses from neighboring neurons leads to the activation of metabotropic glutamate receptors. This allows for calcium influx which consequently engages machinery for protein synthesis and permanently changes postsynaptic neurons [34].

3. Microbiota gut brain axis and stroke

Gut-brain axis has recently been increasingly recognized as one of hallmark biological processes linked with the pathophysiology of stroke [35]. Gut-brain axis primarily refers to the network of biological connections that link the gastrointestinal tract (GIT) and the central nervous system (CNS), allowing for bidirectional communication between the two [36, 37]. By implication, the bidirectional communication here indicates two-way communication implying that while on hand the brain modulates the regulation of gut activities (top-down signaling); on the other hand, the gut also can regulate the functions of the brain (bottom-up signaling). These regulatory signals between the two are executed through multiple mechanisms, including neural, endocrinal, immunological, and metabolic pathways. The components of the brain that drive gut-brain axis include the hypothalamus, medial prefrontal cortex, nucleus of the solitary tract in the medulla, and amygdala among others [38]. The gastrointestinal components include the intestinal cells and the microbes within the gut termed microbiota. The term gut microbiota refers to complex assembly of microbes residing within the human gastrointestinal tract [39]. The microbes within microbiota community are constituted by extraordinary densities of 100 trillions of microorganisms, including more than 1000 species, of mostly bacteria, but also fungi, archaea, protozoa, and viruses, together with their collective genomes termed microbiome [21, 22]. Because the gut microbiota contributes to the major components involved in gut-brain axis, the term microbiota gut-brain axis is used as an extension to recognize the integral position of gut microbiota in gut-brain axis [40].

Mounting lines of evidence demonstrate that gut microbiota dysbiosis is one of the key causative factors in stroke pathology, and the interaction between stroke and microbiota pathologies is noticeable via microbiota-gut-brain-axis. The term dysbiosis is used to indicate disruption in the balance of composition of gut microbiota towards decreased intestinal biodiversity of beneficial or commensal species and increased pathogenic bacteria species [41]. Under normal circumstances, the composition of intestinal microbiota is in a status of eubiosis, where there's a preponderance of potentially beneficial species such as *Firmicutes* and *Bacteroides* over a very low percentage of potentially pathogenic species such as *Proteobacteria*. This normal balance is critical for health and homeostasis, especially in the brain, and when dysfunctional leads to the development and progression of diseases [42]. For instance, stroke leads to gut microbiota dysbiosis, and this causes dysfunctional gut-brain axis signaling that further amplified neuroinflammation and oxidative stress damage.

Several studies involving human and animal models of stroke have demonstrated gut microbiota dysbiosis involvement in the pathology of stroke. Stanley [43] examined the composition of the mucosal microbiota after stroke in a model of focal cerebral ischemia. This study found that ischemic stroke is associated with microbiota dysbiosis, as well as far-reaching and robust changes to the intestinal mucosal microbiota. Crasper [44] observed the role of bacterial translocation from the gut in post-stroke infection in an animal model of stroke. It was observed from this study that ischemic stroke results in impairment of gut permeability, as well as a marked inducement in gut dysbiosis. Stanley [45] studied whether post-stroke infection originated from commensal bacteria that normally reside in the intestinal tracts. Animal models that had post-stroke lung infection microbiota were observed, the microbes were found to originate from small intestinal microbes by more than 60%, and this was attributed to stroke-induced impairment in gut barrier that allows for intestinal microbiota to reach peripheral tissues.

Haak [46] studied the hypothesis of whether patients diagnosed with acute ischemic stroke and manifest with dysbiosis in gut microbiota composition may change the risk development of post-stroke infections following hospitalization in a case–control study. Outcome of this study revealed a drastic reduction in anaerobic gut bacteria in stroke cases, which is closely associated with post-stroke infection. Boaden [47] performed a case–control study involving patients diagnosed and screened with ischemic stroke to determine the composition of gut microbiota and its important blood metabolite trimethylamine-N-oxide. Ischemic stroke patients were found to have mark dysbiosis in gut microbiota composition with more preponderance of pathogenic microbiome and fewer commensal or beneficial microbiome. This dysbiosis was found to be correlated with the stroke severity. The blood level of trimethylamine-N-oxide was in contrast found to be significantly lower in patients with ischemic stroke. Tan [48] evaluated the gut microbiome and short-chain fatty acids spectrum, as well as their possible relation with the measure of variability in ischemic stroke severities. A mark change in composition of intestinal microbiota was observed among stroke patients when compared with control, specifically depicting deficiency in short-chain fatty acids producing bacteria which become marked with the increasing severity of stroke.

Wang [49] designed a study that sought to determine intestinal flora diversity in patients diagnosed and screened with ischemic stroke, as well as investigate whether the intestinal microflora can be used as a marker for early diagnosis of cerebral infarction. Intestinal flora composition was found to be significantly different between ischemic stroke patients in relative to the healthy control. Intestinal flora composition could be an important indicator for cerebral infarction, and due to the observed positive correlation between serum level apolipoprotein E and Gamma-proteobacteria, the serum level apolipoprotein E holds potential to predict cerebral infarction. Huang [50] carried out a study that aimed to investigate the variability in characteristics of gut microbiota among patients with acute cerebral infarction. It was revealed from this study that the abundance of three bacterial species that were abnormally higher in patients with acute cerebral ischemia in comparison to healthy controls. Yamashiro [51] observed two parameters of gut microbiota, its constituent composition, and organic acid content if they are related with ischemic stroke, and whether there is a relationship that could result in mediating biological processes such as metabolism and inflammation. Findings showed evidence of microbiota dysbiosis among the patients diagnosed with ischemic stroke, this dysbiosis was found to be associated with biological indicators of host inflammation (such as interleukin-6, high sensitivity C-reactive protein, and with white blood cell counts) and metabolism (such as acetic acid, valeric acid, and low-density lipoprotein cholesterol).

Li [52] set out a study to examine the variation in gut microbiota profile between patients diagnosed and screened with ischemic in comparison with healthy controls, and to study if such variation will be associated with the assessed clinical parameters. Patients with cerebral infarction showed dysbiosis in gut microbiota composition. This dysbiosis is related to clinical measures of stroke severity, as bacterial genera that were found to be reduced among stroke patients were negatively associated with stroke severity. Singh [53] carried out a study to determine the mechanism through which post-stroke dysbiosis links with immune response, especially the intestinal immune cells balance. Ischemic stroke was confirmed to induce dysbiosis of microbiota, and this dysbiosis proved to cause alteration in intestinal immune cells balance.

4. The role of gut microbiome in brain plasticity

Table 1 below shows evidence about the influence of gut microbiome on brain plasticity through microbiota gut-brain axis.

There exist various modalities through which gut microbiome can be modulated to complement neuroplasticity with stroke rehabilitation. Development and testing of specific interventions such as probiotics, prebiotics, dietary-based intervention, or

Modification in microbiota gut-brain axis	Observed corresponding effect in brain plasticity process	Reference
Microbiome deficient model in the form in the germ-free (GF) mice compared with conventionally raised counterparts.	Germ-free mice show changes in electrophysiological properties of hippocampal plasticity, which is associated with dendritic signaling and long-term potentiation (LTP), indicating that absence of a microbiome alters basal synaptic efficacy, and inducibility of plasticity in the hippocampus.	[54]
Microbiome distorted germ-free (GF) mice were compared with conventional mice.	Germ-free mice microbiome modulation with probiotics shows changes in the expression of gamma-aminobutyric acid (GABA) in the hippocampus, indicating a potential role in long-term potentiation and memory.	[55]
The gut microbiota was altered by treatment with antibiotic or germ-free (GF) mice.	Microbiota alterations result in changes in transcriptional profiles of excitatory neurons, glia, and other cell types in the prefrontal cortex. These changes were found to have long-lasting effects on neuronal function and learning-related plasticity that subsequently regulate fear extinction behavior.	[56]
Gut microbiota-based distorted model in germ-free (GF) mice and GF mice colonized post weaning (exGF).	Germ-free mice show difference in expression of splicing factor genes in the amygdala, which is able to partially compensate for impairments in neuronal plasticity signaling.	[57]
Gut microbiota-based altered model in germfree (GF) mice, colonized GF mice (ex-GF) were compared with conventionally raised (CON) mice	Germ-free mice display altered transcriptional profile in genes related to cholinergic and dopaminergic neurotransmission in the amygdala (Drd2, Adora2a, Tac1, Chrnra2, and Chat) that have been implicated as crucial for neural activity, synaptic transmission, neurogenesis, and nervous system development.	[58]
Gut microbiota-based distorted models in germ-free mice (GF; microbiota deficient from birth) were compared with conventionally colonized (CC) mice.	Germ-free mice displayed changes in volume and dendritic morphology of the amygdale, hippocampus, and pyramidal neurons, indicating the role of microbiome in neural remodeling.	[59]
Gut microbiota-deficient animal model in the form of germ-free (GF) mice was compared with their conventionally colonized (CC) mice.	Brain-derived neurotrophic factor (BDNF) expression, a pivotal brain neurotropic molecule essential for neurogenesis and neuroplasticity was observed to be severely decreased in germ-free (GF) mice.	[60]
A germ-free (GF) mice that have altered gut microbiota, were compared with specific pathogen-free (SPF) mice with normal gut microbiota.	A significant decrease in BDNF mRNA expression was observed in germ-free mice within the hippocampus, amygdala, and cingulate cortex. BDNF signaling mediates neural plasticity processes such as neurogenesis, dendritic arborization, and axonal sprouting.	[61]
Gut microbiota altered model in germ-free Swiss Webster mice were compared with colonized counterparts.	Germ-free (GF) mice show distorted BDNF and c-Fos protein expression in the hippocampus.	[62]

Table 1.
Role of gut microbiome on brain plasticity through microbiota gut-brain axis.

any agent that targets particular gut microbiome metabolites will provide a potential novel strategy for gut microbiome-based intervention in stroke rehabilitation.

5. Mechanism through which microbiome-based interventions could improve stroke recovery and rehabilitation

The potentiality of microbiota gut-brain axis in the pathogenesis and therapeutics of stroke has been also promising in human studies. Guo [17] carried out a case–control study involving acute ischemic stroke patients that were treated with traditional Chinese medicine termed tanhuo decoction (THD). It was observed that THD offers neuroprotection via modulation of microbiota gut-brain axis, where it regulates several gut bacteria to lower microbial metabolites such as lipopolysaccharide (LPS) and trimethylamine N-oxide (TMAO). Zhong [63] examined evidence-based literature the effect of probiotics, as one of the specific entities within microbiome-based interventions in the management of patients with stroke. Probiotics were found to possess enormous potential for clinical applicability in promoting stroke recovery. The various mechanisms through which microbiome-based interventions could improve stroke recovery and rehabilitation are illustrated in **Figure 1** below:

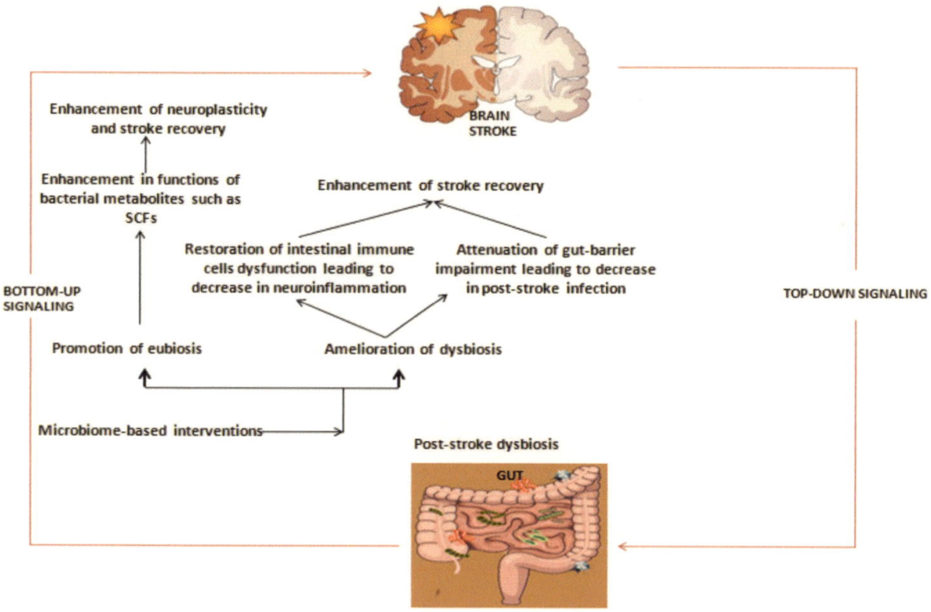

Figure 1.
Schematic illustration of various mechanisms through which microbiome-based interventions could improve stroke recovery and rehabilitation.

6. Conclusion

The role of microbiome-based modulation to mediate brain plasticity through microbiota gut-brain axis is highlighted; this could be fundamental towards translating similar phenomenon in human stroke to promote brain neuroplasticity in complement with post-stroke rehabilitation.

Conflict of interest

The authors declare no conflict of interest.

Author details

Mubarak Muhammad[1*], Rabi'u Musa Isah[2] and Abdurrazak Muhammad[3]

1 Neurorehabilitation Unit, Department of Physiotherapy, Kazaure General Hospital, Kazaure, Jigawa State, Nigeria

2 Department of Physiotherapy, Murtala Muhammad Specialist Hospital, Kano State, Nigeria

3 Department of Chemical Science, School of Science and Information Technology, Skyline University, Nigeria

*Address all correspondence to: mubarakmahmad@yahoo.com

References

[1] Favate S, Younger DS. Epidemiology of ischemic stroke. Neurologic Clinics. 2016;**34**(4):967-980

[2] Feigin VL, Norrving B, Mensah GA. Global burden of stroke. Circulation Research. 2017;**120**(3):439-448

[3] Katan M, Luft A. Global burden of stroke. Seminars in Neurology. 2018;**38**(02):208-211

[4] Muhammad M, Hassan TM. Cerebral damage after stroke: Therole of neuroplasticity as key forrecovery. In: Cerebral Damage after Stroke: The Role of Neuroplasticity as Key for Recovery. London: Intech Open Publishers; 2021. pp. 1-15

[5] Canazza A, Minati L, Boffano C, Parati E, Binks S. Experimental model of brain ischaemia: A review of technique, magnetic resonance imaging, and investigational cell-based therapies. Frontiers in Neurology. 2014;**5**(19):1-15

[6] Elder J, Cortes M, Rykman A, Hill J, Karuppagounder S, Edwards D, et al. The epigenetics of stroke recovery and rehabilitation: From polycomb to histone deacetylases. Neurotherapeutics. 2013;**10**:808-816

[7] Zhao L, Willing A. Enhancing endogenous capacity to repair a stroke damaged brain: An evolving field for stroke research. Progress in Neurobiology. 2018;**164**:5-26

[8] Ekusheva EV, Damulin IV. Post-stroke rehabilitation: Importance of neuroplasticity and sensorimotor integration processes. Neuroscience and Behavioral Physiology. 2015;**45**(5): 594-599

[9] Hara Y. Brain plasticity and rehabilitation in stroke patients. Journal of Nippon Medical School. 2015;**82**:4-13

[10] Murciano-Brea J, Garcia-Montes M, Geuna S, Herrera-Rincon C. Gut microbiota and neuroplasticity. Cell. 2021;**10**:2084

[11] Richards LG, Stewart KC, Woodbury ML, Senesac C, Cauraugh JH. Movement dependent stroke recovery: A systematic review and metaanalysis of TMS and FMRI evidence. Neuropsychologia. 2008;**46**(1):3-11

[12] Szelenberger R, Kostka J, Saluk-Bijak J, Miller E. Pharmacological interventions and rehabilitation approach for enhancing brain selfrepair and stroke recovery. Current Neuropharmacology. 2020;**18**:51-64

[13] Friec AL, Salabert A, Davoust C, Demain B, Vieu C, Vaysse L, et al. Enhancing plasticity of the central nervous system: Drugs, stem cell therapy, and neuro-implants. Neural Plasticity. 2017;**1-9**:2545736

[14] Liu J, Zhang T, Wang Y, Si C, Wang X, Wang R, et al. Baicalin ameliorates neuropathology in repeated cerebral ischemiareperfusion injury model mice by remodeling the gut microbiota. Aging (Albany NY). 2020;**12**(4):3791-3806

[15] Lee J, d'Aigle J, Atadja L, Quaicoe V, Honarpisheh P, Ganesh BP, et al. Gut microbiota-derived short-chain fatty acids promote poststroke recovery in aged mice. Circulation Research. 2020;**127**(4):453-465

[16] Yu X, Zhou G, Shao B, Zhou H, Xu C, Yan F, et al. Gut microbiotadysbiosis

induced by intracerebral hemorrhage aggravates neuroinflammation in mice. Frontiers in Microbiology. 2021;**12**:647304

[17] Guo Q, Jiang X, Ni C, Li L, Chen L, Wang Y, et al. Gut microbiota-related effects of tanhuo decoction in acute ischemic stroke. Oxidative Medicine and Cellular Longevity. 2021:1-18. Article ID: 55969214

[18] Gubert C, Hanna AJ. Plastic brains and gastrointestinal strains: The microbiota-gut-brain axis as a modulator of cellular plasticity and cognitive function (commentary on Darch et al., 2021). European Journal of Neuroscience. 2021;**54**(4):5245-5248

[19] Jandhyala SM, Talukdar R, Subramanyam C, Vuyyuru H, Sasikala M, Reddy ND. Role of the normal gut microbiota. World Journal of Gastroenterology. 2015;**21**(29):8787-8803

[20] Sender R, Fuchs S, Milo R. Revised estimates for the number of human and bacteria cells in the body. PLoS Biology. 2016;**14**(8):e1002533

[21] Brandscheid C, Schuck F, Reinhardt S, Schäfer K, Pietrzik C, Grimm M, et al. Altered gut microbiome composition and tryptic activity of the 5xFAD Alzheimer's mouse model. Journal of Alzheimers Disease. 2017;**56**:775-788

[22] Fang P, Kazmi SA, Jameson KG, Hsiao EY. The microbiome as a modifier of neurodegenerative disease risk. Cell Host & Microbe. 2020;**28**:201-222

[23] Spychala MS, Venna VR, Jandzinski M, Doran S, Durgan DJ, Ganesh BP, et al. Age-related changes in the gut microbiota influence systemic inflammation and stroke outcome. Annals of Neurology. 2018;**84**:23-36

[24] Winek K, Engel O, Koduah P, Heimesaat MM, Fischer A, Bereswill S, et al. Depletion of cultivatable gut microbiota by broad-spectrum antibiotic pretreatment worsens outcome after murine stroke. Stroke. 2016;**47**:1354-1363

[25] Tang W, Zhu H, Feng Y, Guo R, Wan D. The impact of gut microbiota disorders on the blood-brain barrier. Infection and Drug Resistance. 2020;**13**:3351-3363

[26] Dewey HM, Sherry LJ, Collier JM. Stroke rehabilitation 2007: What should it be? International Journal of Stroke. 2007;**2**(3):191Y200

[27] Hurdowar A, Graham ID, Bayley M, Harrison M, Wood-Dauphinee S, Bhogal S. Quality of stroke rehabilitation clinical practice guidelines. Journal of Evaluation in Clinical Practice. 2007;**13**:657-664

[28] Quinn TJ, Paolucci S, Sunnerhagen KS, Sivenius J, Walker MF, Toni D, et al. Evidence-based stroke rehabilitation: An expanded guidance document from the european stroke organisation (ESO) guidelines for management of ischaemic stroke and transient ischaemic attack 2008. Journal of Rehabilitation Medicine. 2009;**41**:99-111

[29] Samir R, Belagaje MD. Stroke rehabilitation. Review. Continuum (Minneap Minn). 2017;**23**(1):238-253

[30] Kleim JA, Jones TA. Principles of experience-dependent neural plasticity: Implications for rehabilitation after brain damage. Journal of Speech, Language, and Hearing Research. 2008;**51**:S225-S239

[31] Warraich Z, Kleim JA. Neural plasticity: The biological substrate

for neurorehabilitation. PM&R. 2010;**2**:S208-S219

[32] Hosp JA, Luft AR. Cortical plasticity during motor learning and recovery after ischemic stroke. Neural Plasticity. 2011;**2011**:871296

[33] Vida D, Sandra M, Raphael B. Neuroplasticity. Periodicum Biologorum. 2014;**116**(2):209-211

[34] Kotaleski JH, Blackwell KT. Modelling the molecularmechanisms of synaptic plasticity using systems biology approaches. Nature Reviews Neuroscience. 2010;**11**(4):239-251

[35] Nobile V, Giardina S, Puoci F. The effect of a probiotic complex on the gut-brain axis: A translational study. Neuropsychobiology. 2021:1-11. PMID: 34515196

[36] García-Cabrerizo R, Carbia C, O'Riordan KJ, Schellekens H, Cryan JF. Microbiota-gut-brain axis as a regulator of reward processes. Journal of Neurochemistry. 2021;**00**:1-30

[37] Socała K, Doboszewska U, Szopa A, Serefko A, Włodarczyk M, Zielinska A, et al. The role of microbiota-gut-brain axis in neuropsychiatric and neurological disorders. Pharmacological Research. 2021;**172**:105840

[38] Browning KN, Travagli RA. Central nervous system control of gastrointestinal motility and secretion and modulation of gastrointestinal functions. Comprehensive Physiology. 2014;**4**:1339-1368

[39] Morki S, Butler M, Holl A, Cryan JF, Dinan TG. Probiotics and the microbiota-gut-brain axis: Focus on psychiatry. Current Nutrition Reports. 2020;**9**:171-182

[40] Peterson CT. Dysfunction of the microbiota-gut-brain axis in neurodegenerative disease: The promise of therapeutic modulation with prebiotics, medicinal herbs, probiotics, and symbiotics. Journal of Evidence-Based Integrative Medicine. 2020;**25**: 1-19

[41] Salami M. Interplay of good bacteria and central nervous system: Cognitive aspects and mechanistic considerations. Frontiers in Neuroscience. 2021; **15**:613120

[42] Aizawa E, Tsuji H, Asahara T, Takahashi T, Teraishi T, Yoshida S, et al. Possible association of Bifidobacterium and lactobacillus in the gutmicrobiota of patients with major depressive disorder. Journal of Affective Disorders. 2016;**202**:254-257

[43] Stanley D, Moore RJ, Wong CHY. An insight into intestinal mucosal microbiota disruption after stroke. Scientific Reports. 2018;**8**:568

[44] Crapser J, Ritzel R, Verma R, Venna VR, Liu F, Chauhan A, et al. Ischemic stroke induces gut permeability and enhances bacterial translocation leading to sepsis in aged mice. Aging (Albany NY). 2016;**8**(5):1049

[45] Stanley D, Mason LJ, Mackin KE, Srikhanta YN, Lyras D, Prakash MD, et al. Translocation and dissemination of commensal bacteria in post-stroke infection. Nature Medicine. 2016;**22**(11):1277-1284

[46] Haak BW, Westendorp WF, van Engelen TSR, Brands X, Brouwer MC, Vermeij J, et al. Disruptions of anaerobic gut bacteria are associated with stroke and post-stroke infection: A prospective case-control study. Translational Stroke Research. 2021;**12**:581-592

[47] Boaden E, Lyons M, Singhrao SK, Dickinson H, Leathley M, Lightbody CE, et al. Oral flora in acute stroke patients: A prospective exploratory observational study. Gerodontology. 2017;**34**(3): 343-356

[48] Tan C, Wu Q, Wang H, Gao X, Xu R, Cui Z, et al. Dysbiosis of gut microbiota and short-chain fatty acids in acute ischemic stroke and the subsequent risk for poor functional outcomes. Journal of Parenteral and Enteral Nutrition. 2021;**45**(3):518-529

[49] Wang W, Li X, Yao X, Cheng X, Zhu Y. The characteristics analysis of intestinal microecology on cerebral infarction patients and its correlation with apolipoprotein E. Medicine. 2018;**97**(41):e12805

[50] Huang L, Wang T, Wu Q, Dong X, Shen F, Liu D, et al. Analysis of microbiota in elderly patients with acute cerebral infarction. Peer J. 2019;7:e6928

[51] Yamashiro K, Tanaka R, Urabe T, Ueno Y, Yamashiro Y, Nomoto K, et al. Gut dysbiosis is associated with metabolism and systemic inflammation in patients with ischemic stroke. PLoS One. 2017;**12**(2):e0171521

[52] Li H, Zhang X, Pan D, Liu Y, Yan X, Tang Y, et al. Dysbiosis characteristics of gut microbiota in cerebral infarction patients. Translational Neuroscience. 2020;**11**(1):124-133

[53] Singh V, Roth S, Llovera G, Sadler R, Garzetti D, Stecher B, et al. Microbiota dysbiosis controls the neuroinflammatory response after stroke. Journal of Neuroscience. 2016;**36**(28):7428-7440

[54] Darch HT, Collins MK, O'Riordan KJ, Cryan JF. Microbial memories: Sex-dependent impact of the gut microbiome on hippocampal plasticity. European Journal of Neuroscience. 2021;**54**(4):5235-5244

[55] Mao JH, Kim YM, Zhou YX, Hu D, Zhong C, Chang H, et al. Genetic and metabolic links between the murine microbiome and memory. Microbiome. 2020;**8**(1):53

[56] Chu C, Murdock MH, Jing D, Won TH, Chung H, Kressel AM, et al. The microbiota regulate neuronal function and fear extinction learning. Nature. 2019;**574**:543-548

[57] Stilling RM, Moloney GM, Ryan FJ, Hoban AE, Bastiaanssen TFS, Shanahan F, et al. Social interaction-induced activation of rna splicing in the amygdala of microbiome-deficient mice. eLife. 2018;7:e33070

[58] Hoban AE, Stilling RM, Moloney G, Shanahan F, Dinan TG, Clarke G, et al. The microbiome regulates amygdale dependent fear recall. Molecular Psychiatry. 2018;**23**:1134-1144

[59] Luczynski P, Whelan SO, O'Sullivan C, Clarke G, Shanahan F, Dinan TG, et al. Adult microbiota-deficient mice has distinct dendritic morphological changes: Differential effects in the amygdala and hippocampus. The European Journal of Neuroscience. 2016;**44**:2654-2666

[60] Clarke G, Grenham S, Scully P, Fitzgerald P, Moloney RD, Shanahan F, et al. The microbiome gut-brain axis during early life regulates the hippocampal serotonergic system in a sex-dependent manner. Molecular Psychiatry. 2013;**18**:666-673

[61] Heijtz RD, Wang S, Anuar F, Qian Y, Björkholm B, Samuelsson A, et al. Normal gut microbiota modulates brain development and behavior. Proc. Natl. Acad. Sci. USA. 2011;**108**:3047-3052

[62] Gareau MG, Wine E, Rodrigues DM, Cho JH, Whary MT, Philpott DJ, et al. Bacterial infection causes stress-induced memory dysfunction in mice. Gut. 2011;**60**(3):307-317

[63] Zhong D, Li L, Ma R, Deng Y. The effect of probiotics in stroke treatment. Evidence-based Complementary and Alternative Medicine. 2021;**2021**:1-10

Chapter 7

Non-invasive Brain Stimulation Post Stroke

Fahad Somaa

Abstract

Stroke is the second most common cause of death and dementia and the first most common cause of disability in developed nations. Tissue in the penumbra may be salvaged by reperfusion treatment using recombinant tissue plasminogen activator or thrombectomy with a stent retriever, which improves the ultimate neurological prognosis. However, because of the limited therapeutic window of 6 hours, it is only available to 5–10% of the community. Non-invasive brain stimulation (NIBS) has recently gotten a lot of interest for its potential involvement in stroke recovery. When used correctly, NIBS methods employ electrical and magnetic stimulation to modify the excitability of deep brain tissue without harming it. This may result in long-term neuroplastic modifications. Based on different protocols, stimulation to the cerebral cortex can be either excitatory or inhibitory. This has led to NIBS being used therapeutically to alleviate depression. In recent years, stroke patients have been studied to see whether NIBS has therapeutic benefits on cognitive skills.

Keywords: stroke, brain stimulation, non-invasive brain stimulation, rehabilitation, plasticity

1. Introduction

Stroke is the world's second leading cause of death and the third leading cause of disability [1]. Stroke survivors may experience a variety of disabilities that require temporary or long-term assistance. It has a major impact on the patient, their family, the economy of the country, and the world economy [2]. The burden of stroke-related damage is expected to rise in the following decades as the population ages. Even though the death rate from stroke has reduced, the incidence of stroke has not, increasing the number of stroke survivors [3].

Even if people with this condition survive the acute period of their illness, they may have long-term physical and psychological consequences. After the first stroke, the quality of life and health are significantly reduced due to post-stroke impairment [4]. It is still difficult to regain arm and hand function after a stroke, despite stroke rehabilitation methods showing some promise. Due to the increase in the incidence of strokes in 2030 and inadequate facilities offering reperfusion treatments within the small therapeutic window, novel approaches to promote spontaneous brain plasticity are needed [5]. Post-lesional brain plasticity after stroke may be helpful or "adaptive," or harmful or "maladaptive," which hinders neurological rehabilitation [6].

Individuals may have considerable dysfunction due to cognitive impairment after a stroke. Memory loss, attention problems, executive and behaviour issues are the most common symptoms seen. After conducting a nationwide epidemiological cohort study on the population and prevalence of chronic brain damage, researchers found that memory impairment (90%), attention disturbance (82%), and executive function impairments were the most frequent cognitive symptoms (75%). Injury mechanisms, demographics, and social variables all impact the intensity and range of cognitive symptoms. Research suggests that 42–92% of patients in the acute phase have attention deficit disorder, and 24–51% have symptoms after leaving acute care. According to recent research, 23–55% of stroke survivors experience memory problems within 3 months, while 11–31% experience memory impairment a year after their stroke. This percentage is comparable in the traumatic brain injury (TBI) group (25%). When people suffer from Unilateral Spatial Neglect (USN) [7], they have trouble orienting themselves or responding or reporting stimuli that emerge on the side opposite the lesion. Stroke patients are more likely than the average population to develop USN. As a result of these cognitive difficulties, rehabilitation efforts are severely hampered, as is returning to work. Cognitive rehabilitation is primarily concerned with making positive changes in a person's day-to-day life. Instead, cognitive rehabilitation relies on learning compensatory techniques and strategies that have an impact on cognitive function [8]. Several systematic evaluations have looked at how well people recover cognitively after a stroke or traumatic brain injury [9].

In addition to invasive treatments, there has been an increase in interest in examining the influence of non-invasive cortical stimulation on the rehabilitation process [3]. Neuromodulatory non-invasive brain stimulation (NIBS) approaches are being tested to improve motor function following a stroke. Neuromodulation aims to improve adaptively or reduce maladaptive post-stroke reorganisation processes [10].

The idea behind NIBS came from Faraday's law of induction when, in the 1980s, some researchers stimulated specific areas of the brain using a pulsed magnetic field and noticed changes in the neuronal firing and impulse conduction. Barker et al. demonstrated the first example of transcranial magnetic stimulation (TMS) [11].

Prior to that, electroconvulsive therapy (ECT) to treat severe depression had already been in use since the 1940s. Further studies led to the knowledge that TMS can change the balance between excitation and inhibition leading to speculation that it might be useful in treating conditions such as Parkinson's disease. However, it was not until the 1990s that specific stimulators were developed that could deliver repetitive impulses to the brain. This lead to the development of a technique called transcranial direct-current stimulation (tDCS) [12, 13].

Transcranial magnetic stimulation (TMS) and transcranial direct-current stimulation (tDCS) have been studied for their effects on motor, sensory, and cognitive skills in stroke patients [3].

TMS can change function and enhance or reduce activity in cortical areas depending on stimulation frequency, duration, coil form, and magnetic field strength. The effects of repeated transcranial magnetic stimulation (rTMS) on cortical excitability can linger up to 2 hours after the stimulation cycle has ended. From minutes to 1 to 2 hours, tDCS can increase or decrease excitability in the stimulated region. Unlike TMS, tDCS appears to modify the activation of sodium- and calcium-dependent channels, as well as NMDA receptor function, causing LTP and LTD-like alterations (**Figure 1**) [15, 16].

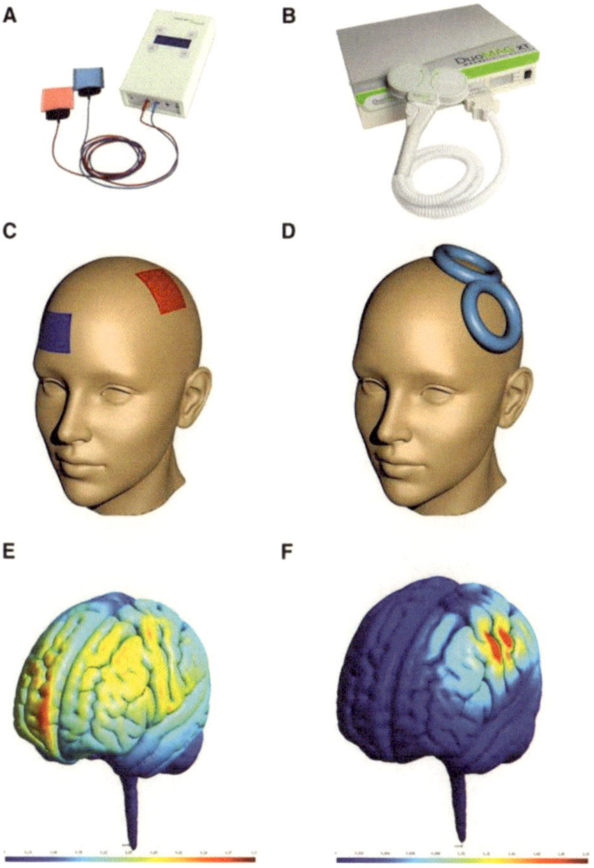

Figure 1.
Examples of commercial (A) transcranial direct-current stimulation and (B) transcranial magnetic stimulation equipment, (C, D) coil/electrode montage over the motor cortex, and (D, E) maps of electrical fields generated [14].

1.1 Brain plasticity after stroke

Cortical plasticity refers to the brain's capacity to change how it functions as a consequence of new learning. In other words "plasticity" refers to any changes in brain organisation as a result of repeated exposure to a stimulus. The term "synaptic plasticity" refers to the ability of synapses to change their strength over time. A single synapse houses all of the plasticity's manifestations. Both short-term synaptic plasticity and long-term synaptic plasticity have been documented, indicating that synaptic transmission may be boosted or decreased in different time periods [17]. A mechanism known as LTP has been extensively explored when it comes to learning and memory. However, brain damage has been linked to plasticity. That is all it says about the processes at work; it does not explain how the brain may modify its functional and structural structure (both histologically and anthropologically) in the wake of injury and make better use of what is left. The excitability of neuronal networks close and far from the affected region is altered by a stroke. There is less or greater positive plasticity in people who do not fully heal from their injuries. Activity-dependent rebuilding and synaptic strengthening are two pathways for plasticity. Brain-derived nerve factor (BDNF) increases glutamate release and synaptic activity over time. According to animal studies, after a stroke, there is a short window of neuroplasticity during which the most significant advances in recovery may be made. Identifying the processes involved in post-stroke healing and optimising their promotion in each person is the problem.

Another problem is that opposite effects occur at the same time. Tonic inhibition through GABA overexpression is seen in the acute phase of the peri-infarct region. Neuroprotective method to prevent excitotoxicity as well as neuronal death has been hypothesised. Increasing behavioural recovery by blocking GABAergic activity for 1 month might be beneficial. TMS may detect this drop-in activity in the acute period in the patient. The idea was developed over two decades ago, works by delivering a high-intensity electric current through a coil to activate the cortex. For a duration of 0.3–1 ms, a magnetic field of 2–2.5 Tesla is generated by a microsecond-long discharge. A coil is positioned on the scalp to reach the cortex, and the coil creates a magnetic current. An electromagnetic field is formed inside the brain, which dissipates after 3 cm, according to the Faraday principle. This electric field depolarizes neurons in the brain beneath the coil, either directly through an axon hillock or indirectly through depolarizing interneurons [18].

The result of using TMS on the motor cortex is an involuntary contralateral muscular contraction. The magnitude of this motor-evoked potential (MEP) is connected to the number of neurons that have responded to the stimulation, and the latency is a technique to determine that how long it takes for inspiration to generate an MEP. Stroke survivors are on a follow-up of up to 1 year using the following prognostic criteria—the persistence of a motor-evoked potential (MEP) after stimulating the affected hemisphere, which is an excellent predictor of recovery. In contrast, hypo excitability showing lack of response is an indicator of poor functional outcome. However, a condition known as “diaschisis” might result from a unilateral brain injury in which brain regions are affected distant from the lesion site. This term was first used in 1914 by von Monakow. The consequences of a localised brain lesion on physically distant but functionally related regions are discussed [19]. It was initially a clinical notion, but several functional imaging modalities that indicate a change in blood flow to the brain in targeted regions make it possible to display cerebellar diaschisis and transcallosal diaschisis on contralateral cortical regions. A deafferentation mechanism in which the wounded cortex prevents the healthy target structure from being activated is the principle at work (or injured subcortical area). According to Roy and Sherrington’s neurovascular coupling hypothesis, this activation may be either excitatory or inhibitory, affecting the metabolism and local blood flow [20].

The existence of a cortico-cerebellar diaschisis during the acute phase of stroke was related to a worse clinical prognosis after 2 months. Through the corpus callosum, the inter-hemispheric route is highly inhibited. Healthy brains have balanced interhemispheric inhibition, meaning that neither hemisphere is a more significant “inhibitor” than another. Neurovascular coupling theory says that after an infarct on one side, increased cerebral blood flow in the contralateral identical region corresponds to greater activity in that region. This was associated with the most severe impairments, which was surprising. As a result, the contralateral hemisphere continues to impose its inhibitory tone on ischemic hypoactivity, adding to the neurological deficit’s rapid progression. As previously stated, the stroke and the overwhelming imbalanced inhibitory impulse from the better and healthier contralateral hemisphere would cause the ipsilateral ischemic cortex to become doubly impaired.

As early as the first week following a stroke, there is evidence of an unbalanced interhemispheric inhibition. Two types of intracortical inhibitory circuits may be studied using TMS paired-pulse protocols—those that are mediated by GABA-A and those by GABA-B.TMS was utilised to discover predictive markers in an investigation of 10 stroke patients who were followed up for 6 months. Recovery is linked to the ipsilateral cortico-spinal pathways of the impacted hemisphere's comparable integrity in the acute period (as measured by MEP and motor threshold). In both hemispheres, however, recovery is connected to the creation of alternative neural networks as measured with short-term and long-term intracortical inhibition [21].

The contralateral hemisphere appeared to be more significant in major infarcts than in mild infarcts in this small sample. However, extrapolating results to all stroke patients is problematic because of the limited sample and various abnormalities (in the anterior and posterior circulation area, cortical or subcortical). The hemiparetic impairment is worsened in animal tests when the lidocaine is applied to the unaffected hemisphere 4 weeks before the injection, and the middle cerebral artery is closed. This is particularly true if significant lesions are created. As a result, whereas an interhemispheric imbalance is harmful during the acute phase, it is helpful throughout the healing period [22].

Physical medicine and rehabilitation facilities increasingly utilise constraint-induced treatment, which is a direct result of these findings. Forcing a person with cerebral palsy to use one limb while forcing the healthy limb to be inactive is the idea. Two things happen—the stroke-related contralateral main motor cortex region is less active, minimising its inhibitory transcallosal and harmful influence on the ischemic hemisphere, while the ipsilateral hemisphere is overactive. For example, in a meta-analysis of controlled trials of "constraint-induced therapy," researchers found that the paretic limb improved steadily over time [23]. Still, they could not develop an exact treatment plan because of the wide variety of treatment protocols utilised and the limited number of participants. There was a remarkable correlation between the clinical improvement and the two-fold increase in the excitability characteristics of the damaged hemisphere as evaluated by TMS.

2. Nibs

2.1 rTMS

The brain is stimulated by rTMS, also known as repetitive transcranial magnetic stimulation. It includes a continuous sequence of pulses or periodic cycles that alter corticospinal reactivity and processes that might be comparable to LTD or LTP. A further week or two is spent repeating the daily exposure of the exact location for 20 minutes. Pacing has an impact on the outcome. Cortical excitability rises with high-frequency stimulation (i.e., >3 Hz) and decreases with a low-frequency stimulus (i.e., less than 1 Hz) [24].

A conscious patient may quickly and painlessly operate this device. Involuntary contralateral muscle contractions, which may be captured as an MEP, indicate exactly where the coil should be placed over the main motor cortex (M1). A real-time neuro-navigation in conjunction with a patient's own cerebral MRI is indicated as soon as the targeted stimulated region is outside M1. The degree of spatial/temporal resolution through this technique is excellent. However, large and costly equipment is needed, and it cannot be done at the patient's bedside [25].

Repetitive transcranial magnetic stimulation (rTMS) underwent modifications to create theta-burst stimulation. It uses 50 Hz pulses delivered in three-pulse bursts, separated by a five-pulse gap. Intermittent theta-burst stimulation uses TBS trains lasting 2 s that are repeated every 10 s, increasing excitability. Continuous theta-burst stimulation, on the other hand, uses TBS trains lasting 20–40 seconds to reduce excitability in the cortex (**Figure 2**).

2.2 tDCS

DCS of the brain in tDCS is more of a neuromodulator than anything else. It is a lot smaller and more portable electrophysiological equipment that may be used at the patient's bedside. Weak polarising direct current is delivered into the brain by two large electrodes on the head. To modify the threshold of cortical neurons and the intrinsic excitability of the cortex, a direct current source (0.5–2 mA) is used. At the same time, the active electrode is placed over the desired location. Network excitability is polarity-dependent—anodal stimulation raises it, whereas cathodal stimulation lowers it. TDCS is also more convenient to utilise in conjunction with behavioural tasks or during physical and occupational therapy due to its small size (**Figures 3** and **4**) [29].

2.3 NIBS for stroke patients

More than 1400 papers have been published thus far on NIBS in humans, with 230 of those papers focusing on stroke-related issues. Mostly, they are concerned with assessing upper-limb motor function, with speech impairments coming in second.

When we look at animal studies there are comparatively little preclinical non-human data on NIBS. The reasons for this are (a) the unavailability of small-sized equipment and (b) ethical issues regarding animal safety. The first animal study for NIBS was conducted in 1990 on rats. Thereafter, a number of studies were conducted on animal models to study the effects of NIBS in Alzheimer's disease, depression,

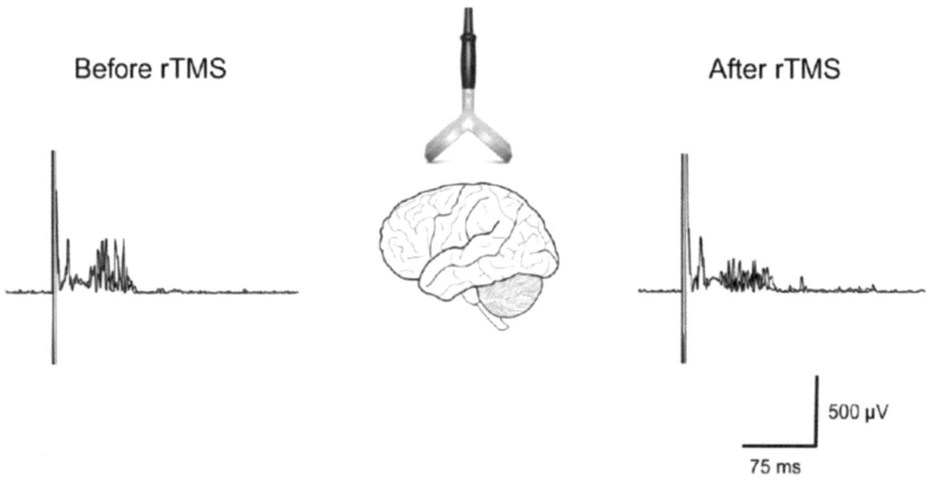

Figure 2.
Blink reflex recordings in a male patient with spinal cord injury before and after rTMS over the vertex [26].

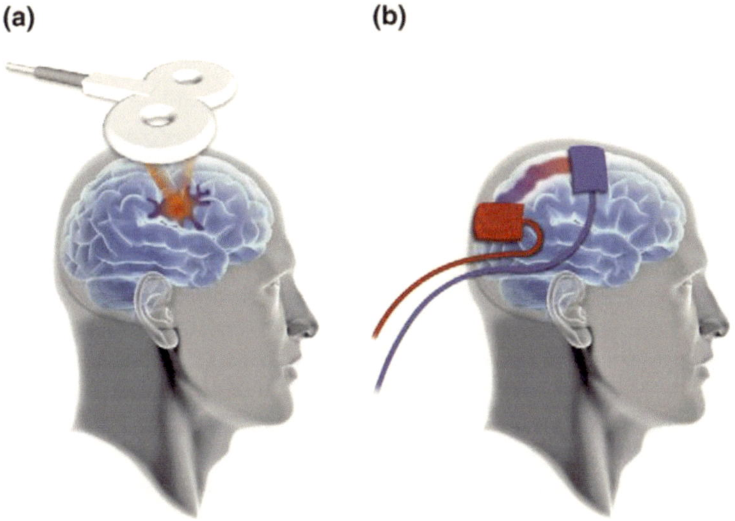

Figure 3.
(a) TMS, (b) tACS application of alternating current through an electrode [27].

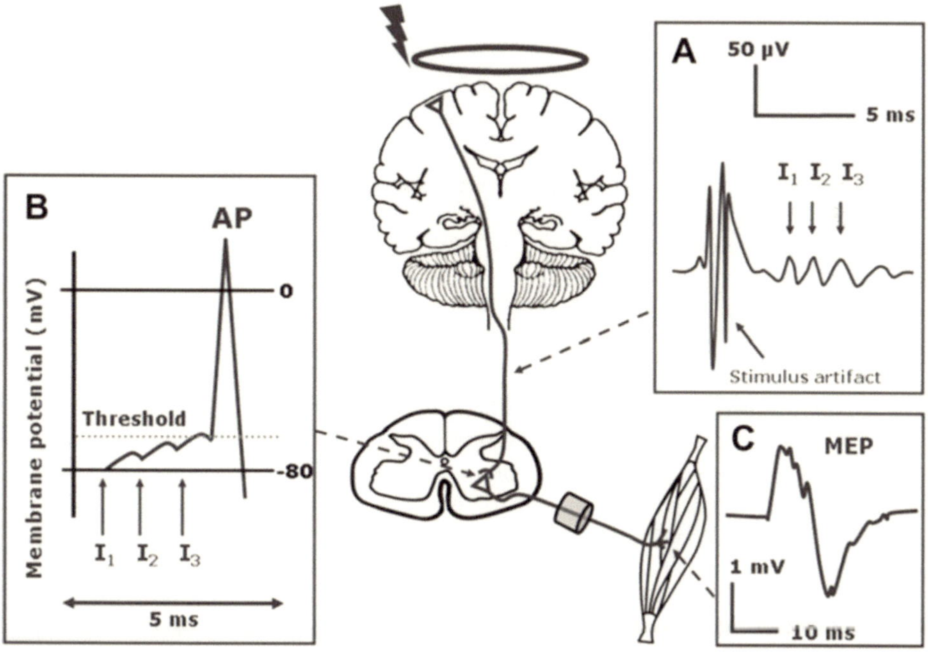

Figure 4.
TMS induced motor evoked potential [28]. Neurophysiological basis of the motor evoked potential (MEP). (A) TMS-induced activation of the corticospinal neurons with a predominant contribution by late Indirect waves (I waves). and (B) Temporo-spatial summation at the cortico-motoneuronal synapses (C) Motor evoked potential.

epilepsy, Huntington's disease, and stroke. These studies demonstrated positive effects of NIBS on neurorepair, particularly improved motor and cognitive performance. The results of these studies have contributed significantly towards the development of NIBS strategies and protocols [30, 31].

NIBS has been linked to post-stroke aphasia, apraxia, attention, gait abnormalities, and coordination deficits. NIBS stroke treatment techniques were created to improve "adaptive" plasticity and combat "maladaptive" plasticity [22].

After a left hemisphere stroke, aphasia is a frequent side effect. In the past 10 to 15 years, advances in neuroimaging have shown two distinct patterns—Patients with minor left hemisphere lesions are more likely to engage perilesional areas, while individuals with larger ones in the left hemisphere are more likely to recruit homotopic areas mostly in the right. By activating the lesional and contralesional regions of the brain, many non-invasive brain stimulation treatments have been utilised to assist patients to recover from a stroke. Most of these brain stimulation investigations focused on blocking homotopic areas in the right posterior IFG (triangular portion) to effect a supposedly disinhibited right inferior frontal gyrus. In other experiments, the contralesional (right) frontotemporal area or sections of the intact left IFG and perilesional areas have also been stimulated with anodal or excitatory tDCS to increase speech-motor output. Since it provides the cornerstone for motor cortex stimulation research, the interhemispheric disinhibition notion also applies to the language system [32].

2.4 Use of combined treatments methods

Whether NIBS combined with rigorous physical therapy, constraint-induced treatment, robot therapy, or EMG-triggered functional neuromuscular stimulation has any added benefits, remains debatable. NIBS can be used with rTMS or tDCS, but there are no data to support it. This failure remains mysterious. To begin with, it is possible that following the initial process there will be a ceiling effect. The other theory is that the adjuvant treatment has an inhibitory impact rather than a priming effect created by the initial surgery. For this to be adequately understood, it must be viewed in conjunction with the concept of metaplasticity—that is, the ability of activity-dependent synaptic plasticity to be influenced by prior activity at synapses, thereby shifting the criterion for LTP and LTD induction—as well as the concept of homeostatic plasticity, which allows neurons as well as circuits to maintain stability despite synaptic instabilities. Therefore, NIBS may have opposing and invalidating effects on the motor task depending on when it is used (prior, during, or just after neurorehabilitation). Motor learning and NIBS may interact differently depending on when it is administered. More profound knowledge of this interaction is needed to determine whether or not it impacts the synaptic state [33].

There is a larger risk of epilepsy during the acute period of recovery. Therefore early research remains focused on whether or not rTMS could be used to assess the inhibition of the contralateral, unaffected main motor region 3–12 months following stroke. One-time (30-minute) or repeated (20–30-minute) treatments were given to patients with acute ischemic stroke for five working days. Chronic stroke patients were treated with 10 Hz excitatory rTMS, and their brain activity was monitored immediately after the treatment. There were just 10–20 patients in each of the first four investigations. According to research, higher frequencies (3 Hz) were shown to be beneficial in the acute phase, 10 days following the start of the stroke. They found no extra advantage to delivering a greater primary cortex excitation (10 vs. 3 Hz) when contrasting two high-frequency impulses. The treated groups had altered MEP and motor thresholds, as well [18].

These investigations were modest (even in the more extensive trials, 20% of patients were lost to follow-up), although the infarcts were clinically and radiographically homogenous, with subcortical infarcts being the most common. Researchers used a randomised control experiment known as a "crossover study" to assign participants to either receive actual or "sham" stimulation, followed by a 1-week washout period or be randomly assigned to get either one or the other.

Throughout most crossover experiments, patients received one rTMS treatment and one sham session separated by 1 week. The sequence of the trials was chosen at random, and most of the time, the assessment focused on measuring handgrip power or pinching power and velocity. When particularly examined, the rTMS effect had vanished after 30 minutes, indicating that it had no impact on the next session's outcomes.

Because the device is less costly and simpler to use than rTMS, tDCS offers great potential. tDCS has been found to extend the time it takes for patients to recover from motor impairments when used repeatedly. To combat extremely high levels of interhemispheric inhibition via the contralesional M1 and reverse the ipsilesional hypoexcitability, stimulation paradigms such as cathodal stimulation of the undamaged hemisphere and anodal stimulation of the afflicted hemisphere have been proposed. Repetitive transcranial magnetic stimulation (rTMS) has been used mostly in the chronic phase of illness for repeated tDCS sessions. For example, it was found that compared to sham tDCS, cathodal tDCS of the unaffected hemisphere enhanced hand motor performance, which was assessed by a blinded Jebsen Taylor Hand function test. The effects of cathodal tDCS applied 5 days in a row persisted for at least 2 weeks. Lindenberg et al. investigated tDCS stimulation (cathodal stimulation in the unaffected hemisphere and anodal stimulation in the afflicted hemisphere) in 20 chronic stroke patients who were also receiving physical and occupational therapy (with a follow-up of more than 5 months) [34]. When compared to placebo, real stimulation resulted in a greater improvement in motor function (+21% for Fugl-Meyer and 19% for Wolf Motor Function test scores), and this improvement lasted at least 1 week following the treatment. It was shown that in the group that received actual stimulation, the ipsilesional primary and premotor cortexes were more active during timed movements of the afflicted limb [35].

3. Stimulation protocols using reorganisation models as a base

Before now, most NIBS procedures were built on the interhemispheric competitive concept, which holds that the healthy hemisphere suppresses the injured hemisphere excessively. This model-based strategy is widely employed in recent and continuing clinical studies, despite being typically useless at the collective level. The reliability of this concept has been called into doubt, particularly in seriously damaged individuals, and an alternate model, the vicariation model, has been proposed. According to this model [22] when one of the brain's hemispheres is impaired, the other makes up for it by performing better and resulting in an adaptive system rather than a maladaptive one.

The bimodal-balance recovery model combines these previously disparate theories, allowing us to get closer to personalised treatment. Assume that a patient is best served by the inter-hemispheric competition or vicariation model. It uses a metric known as "structural reserve" in this situation, which is defined as the integrity of white matter motor pathways. Patients with a strong structural reserve have a maladaptive over-activation of the undamaged hemisphere; patients with poor structural reserve have a compensating over-activation [36]. The fact that patients with extensive brain damage, who are thought to have a limited structural reserve, have inferior results when inhibitory NIBS protocols are administered to their undamaged hemispheres supports this approach, stressing the need to change "one-size-fits-all" NIBS protocols. However, whether clinical and imaging parameters may serve as good substitutes for structural reserve has not been answered. Much research has looked at these factors' capacity to predict stroke outcome, but the strongest evidence comes from those studies [37]. Using diffusion tensor imaging, the fractional anisotropy for white matter tracts is routinely employed to quantify white matter integrity. Although stroke prognosis may be accurately predicted with a strong predictive biomarker, this is not always the case for responding to certain NIBS paradigms. Prognostic biomarkers could be a good place to start, but they must be verified to show their unique function and relative relevance in affecting the outcome of NIBS after a stroke reaction. According to two recent promising studies, behavioural assessments like the Action Research Arm Test and the Fugl-Meyer score, together with imaging-based measures of white matter integrity, are predictive of responsiveness to NIBS. As a result of such studies, the bimodal-balance recovery model is given support, as are future studies that will validate these selection biomarkers using clinical and imaging initiatives related to the structural reserve [38].

Methodologically, significant/extensive trials with many individuals and variables are required to build a framework for customising the treatment for each patient using NIBS. Machine learning algorithms would be best suited for analysing such vast volumes of complicated data. Because of the strong association between imaging-based biomarkers and clinical manifestations of stroke, potential models for guiding NIBS therapy do not need to be particularly complicated. Instead, strongly correlated steps can be whittled down to factors of a lower dimension that describe a significant amount of variability.

4. Connectivity across the entire nervous system

Stroke is a widespread illness that affects people throughout the body. After a stroke, the impact of disrupted networks may be felt far and wide, and the formation of new indirect connections is the fundamental mechanism regulating these effects [39]. Individual stroke recovery is linked to alterations in long-range connections between different brain areas outside of lesions, as well as their regulation throughout time, as studied in resting-state functional MRI in whole-brain. Alterations best describe a single patient in numerous functional networks, which are common in strokes. Since both stroke connectivity and NIBS protocol changes have primarily been examined in the setting of isolated networks, these variables are likely to have contributed to the documented response variability with NIBS. However, this has not been fully explored thus far. It's hard to assume that a single functional network is being addressed in these patients when administering stimulation because of the impact of NIBS on dispersed networks and the notion of stroke as a dispersed disease. Rs-fMRI whole-brain connectivity is ideal for application in patients since it provides information on the functional connectivity of several brain networks in a single task-free scan. A much more accurate model of spontaneous reorganisation following stroke might be developed using this method, and it could be useful in devising personalised stimulation regimes [10]. Connectivity techniques have a methodological disadvantage in that they depend on a prior determination of relatively arbitrary multiple networks. This issue is solved by reducing the number of dimensions in the brain's connections. Areas are grouped in a parametric, gradual way based on their connection patterns using the data-driven technique. Reduced dimensionality of whole-brain linkages may offer a fingerprinting of the connectome at the individual level, reflecting a clearer image of stroke spanning several functional domains. When we used this technique to study stroke lesions, we discovered that the degree of rearrangement that occurred in the first week after stroke was linked to the position of the stroke lesions in space for whole-brain neural systems. We believe that constructing whole-brain connection models will help us better understand the long-term consequences of localised lesions [40].

NIBS reaction prediction using electroencephalogram (EEG) connectivity has shown impressive outcomes. Functional integration modifications to prognostic models of stroke output have added value, so we believe connectivity patterns could be a potential biomarker for NIBS responses in future research. As time goes on, establishing a relationship between a connectome fingerprint and sudden retrieval in several functional domains will be critical and the impact of the connectome fingerprint on clinical reactions to NIBS before stimulation.

5. Neuronal oscillations that are ongoing

A variety of variables may influence response to NIBS, both instantaneous ("state") as well as phenotypic ("trait"). Both may be evaluated using the features of neural oscillations, which indicate the cortex's receptivity to stimulus. You cannot know in advance how someone will react to a stimulation procedure. Even in the absence of disease, the same NIBS procedure might have excitation, inhibiting, or no impacts on motor elicited potentials in different people. One strategy is to time the stimulation to coincide with the most excitable brain states to limit this unpredictability. The findings that pre-stimulus alpha oscillations correlate with TMS response variability, that the intensity of sensorimotor mu oscillations (8–12 Hz over central-parietal electrodes) correlates with the magnitude of motor evoked potentials, and that the synchrony of mu oscillations in contralateral M1 is related to greater inter-hemispheric inhibition, all support the importance of these processes [10]. Current research focuses on NIBS that are "state-dependent."

Subject-specific and highly heritable characteristics of neuronal oscillations characterise immediate cortical responsiveness to NIBS Alpha band (80 Hz) power, and the temporal variation of α- and β-band oscillations are especially relevant here. These findings support the hypothesis that neuronal oscillation features during rest might reflect a phenotypic trait in addition to transitory situations. Healthy people have reasonably good intra-subject reliability for the response to NIBS, which is also strongly heritable. Recently, EEG research found a correlation between healthy people's reaction to paired-pulse TMS and alpha band temporal dynamics before intervention on an individual basis. These findings demonstrate that cortical plasticity is purely genetic, indicating that the brain can be controlled in a trait-like manner [41].

The critical condition is an equilibrium between inhibitory and excitatory that is best for processing information in neural networks. Additionally, critical states are connected with long-range temporal connections (LRTCs) in neuronal oscillation amplitude dynamics. Following a stroke, and various other neuropsychiatric illnesses, LRTCs—which connect to cortical excitability—are prone to be disrupted, as they are in both cases. This suggests that patterns of disruption are associated with spontaneous recovery since the network eventually achieves a compensating equilibrium. Clinically approachable approaches such as resting EEG may be used to quantify the trait-like features of neural oscillations [33].

6. Approaches to NIBS that are new

Recent advancements in NIBS technology are expected to aid in the formulation of more personalised treatment plans. Through multi-locus TMS, it will be possible to move beyond single-area stimulation to target specific muscle groups with different functions in post-stroke motor therapy. Because the coil does not need to be repositioned, this method stimulates many locations with excellent temporal accuracy. With improved induced electrical field modelling, it is possible to forecast exactly what changes will be caused by NIBS on some kind of sub-regional level (for instance, in particular areas of the motor homunculus). Finally, non-invasive stimulation techniques such as transcranial focused ultrasound or temporal interference could be used to target deep brain areas that are inaccessible with TMS and tDCS yet critical for dexterity deficiencies and pathological synergies in stroke [42]. They may help progress NIBS translation while accepting the unavoidable variability of stroke pathophysiology and the discovery and validation of useful biomarkers related to NIBS.

6.1 Side effects and ethical issues regarding NIBS

Minimal side effects, such as transient headache, neck pain, and transient hearing changes, have been reported with the use of NIBS by researchers. However, most of these results are from studies that involved single burst stimulation and knowledge about potential

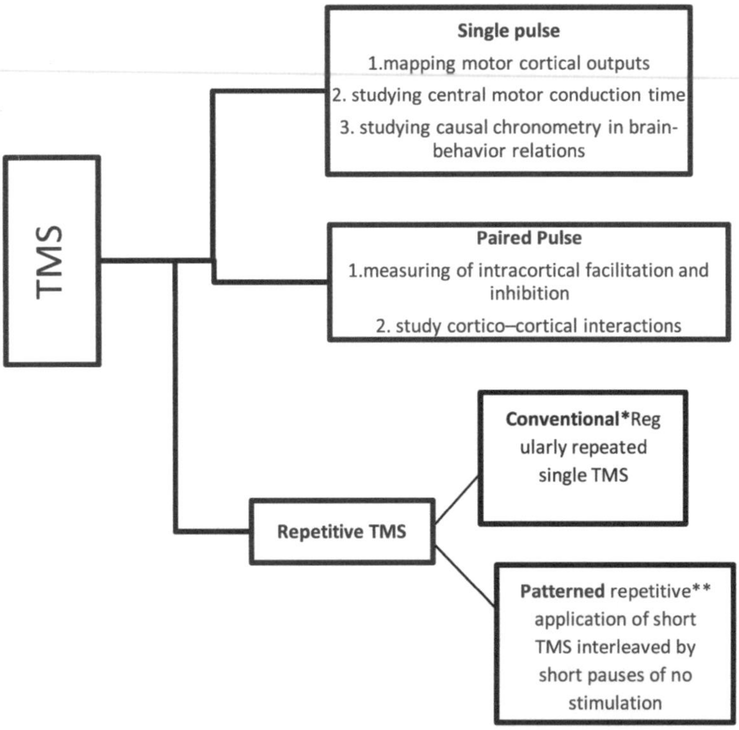

Figure 5.
*Patterns of application of transcranial magnetic stimulation [44]. *convention TMS a. ≤1 Hz stimulation frequency pulses in a continuous train. b. ≥5 Hz stimulation frequency pulses separated by periods of no stimulation (e.g., 1200 pulses at 20 Hz, delivered as 30 trains of 40 pulses (2 s duration) separated by 28 s intertrain intervals. **patterned TMS short bursts of 50 Hz rTMS are repeated at a rate in the theta range (5 Hz).*

	Intensity % of Motor Threshold				
FREQ (Hz)	80-100	100	120	140	160
1	>1800	>1800	360	>50	>50
5	>10	>10	>10	7.6	3.6
10	>5	>5	4.2	1.3	0.9
20	2.05	2.05	1.0	0.35	0.25
25	1.28	1.28	0.4	0.2	0.2

Figure 6.
Maximum safe train duration (seconds) limits [45].

detrimental side effects of repeated stimulation are minimal [43]. An area that poses ethical questions is making the distinction between enhancement and treatment (**Figures 5** and **6**).

In view of ongoing efforts to improve the efficacy of TMS as a technique of inducing persistent changes in brain function, assessing the safety of TMS with neuroimaging becomes extremely important. For therapeutic and research purposes, use of TMS the following three requirements must be kept in mind.

1. Informed consent from the subject or their legal representative

2. Potential benefits must outweigh the risks

3. The subjects chosen must not be socially, physically, or economically vulnerable [44]

6.2 Guidelines for NIBS

There are an infinite number of protocol combinations that can be used. However, it is crucial that careful monitoring of motor, sensory, and cognitive functions be done before, during, and after the intervention.

The resulting growing clinical use of NIBS requires careful guidelines both in terms of equipment and training of the medical staff carrying out NIBS.

In the United States (US), the Food and Drug Administration (FDA) has cleared seven devices for therapeutic TMS in patients of treatment-resistant depression, one device for pre-surgical motor and language cortical mapping, and one device for abortive treatment of migraines. To date, there are no FDA-approved applications of tCS. The FDA takes into account details like coil positioning, output waveform, strength and distribution of the magnetic field safety features of the device.

Currently, there are no requirements or certifications governing a provider's proficiency regarding NIBS before using it. However, it is recommended that all physicians using it undergo training. There are limited programs being offered in some institutes [46].

7. Test results and future trials

Both rTMS and tDCS have been shown to have long-term benefits, with improvements ranging from 10 to 20% based on the literature's upper limb motor performance assessments. In the acute period (6–29 days) high-frequency stimulation of the ipsilaterally affected hemisphere is more effective than low-frequency stimulation of the non-affected, undamaged hemisphere [47].

Stroke-specific adverse effects include moderate headache (2.4%), anxiousness (0.3%), neuro-cardiogenic syncope (0.6%), worsening of pre-existing sleeplessness (0.3%), and local pain at the stimulation site [6]. Adverse events in children and young adults are very similar to those seen in adults—headaches (11.5%), scalp irritation (2.5%), twitching (1.2%), mood swings (1.2%), tiredness (0.9%), tinnitus (0.6%), tingling (11.5%), itchiness (5.8%), redness (4.7%), and scalp irritation (3.1%) have been reported after tDCS protocols [7].

Seizures are the only possible major side effect [48]. Other than stroke peculiarities, certain relevant aspects have been identified from the overall NIBS experience. Even while 0–3.6% of individuals with epilepsy have an epileptic seizure while receiving NIBS, this does not alter the course of their condition. If the antiepileptic plasma level is insufficient, there is a higher incidence of interictal epileptiform discharges (>10/min) and complex temporal seizures are also common (>4/month). Stimulation is followed by a current epileptic seizure (48 hours), and the risk is increased if the epileptogenic region is specifically excited. If there is a family history of epileptic seizures, if the patients receive regular epileptogenic psychotropes, if there is chronic alcohol or opiate abuse, an underpinning neurological disease, severe heart disease, sleep problems, a younger child, or female sex, there is a higher risk of inducing an epileptic seizure in non-epileptic patients [48].

8. Concluding comments

In the literature, the extent of improvement from upper limb motor functional evaluation using rTMS or tDCS is reported to be around 10% and 20%. Clinical trials' results do not match those of meta-analyses, but variability in stroke history, personal susceptibility, outcomes, and a lack of basic understanding of where to administer adjuvant medicines-and the impact of concurrent medications confuse interpretation. As the illness progresses, pharmacological, electrophysiological, or physical adjuvant treatment might potentially improve patient care. Considering the disease's severity, this should favour a patient-tailored strategy more than other techniques.

Author details

Fahad Somaa
Department of Occupational Therapy, King Abdulaziz University, Jeddah, Saudi Arabia

*Address all correspondence to: fsomaa6549@gmail.com

References

[1] Feigin VL, Norrving B, Mensah GA. Global burden of stroke. Circulation Research. 2017;**120**(3):439-448

[2] Luengo-Fernandez R, Violato M, Candio P, Leal J. Economic burden of stroke across Europe: A population-based cost analysis. European Stroke Journal. 2020;**5**(1):17-25

[3] Webster BR, Celnik PA, Cohen LG. Noninvasive brain stimulation in stroke rehabilitation. NeuroRx. 2006; **3**(4):474-481

[4] Abubakar S, Isezuo S. Health related quality of life of stroke survivors: Experience of a stroke unit. International Journal of Biomedical Science: IJBS. 2012;**8**(3):183

[5] Norrving B, Barrick J, Davalos A, Dichgans M, Cordonnier C, Guekht A, et al. Action plan for stroke in Europe 2018-2030. European Stroke Journal. 2018;**3**(4):309-336

[6] Hao Z, Wang D, Zeng Y, Liu M. Repetitive transcranial magnetic stimulation for improving function after stroke. Cochrane Database of Systematic Reviews. 2013;**5**

[7] Swan L. Unilateral spatial neglect. Physical Therapy. 2001;**81**(9):1572-1580

[8] Cicerone KD, Langenbahn DM, Braden C, Malec JF, Kalmar K, Fraas M, et al. Evidence-based cognitive rehabilitation: Updated review of the literature from 2003 through 2008. Archives of Physical Medicine and Rehabilitation. 2011;**92**(4):519-530

[9] Hesse S, Werner C, Schonhardt E, Bardeleben A, Jenrich W, Kirker S. Combined transcranial direct current stimulation and robot-assisted arm training in subacute stroke patients: A pilot study. Restorative Neurology and Neuroscience. 2007;**25**(1):9-15

[10] Ovadia-Caro S, Khalil AA, Sehm B, Villringer A, Nikulin VV, Nazarova M. Predicting the response to non-invasive brain stimulation in stroke. Frontiers in Neurology. 2019;**10**:302

[11] Barker AT, Jalinous R, Freeston IL. Non-invasive magnetic stimulation of human motor cortex. The Lancet. 1985;**325**(8437):1106-1107

[12] Huerta PT, Volpe BT. Transcranial magnetic stimulation, synaptic plasticity and network oscillations. Journal of Neuroengineering and Rehabilitation. 2009;**6**(1):1-10

[13] Dayan E, Censor N, Buch ER, Sandrini M, Cohen LG. Noninvasive brain stimulation: From physiology to network dynamics and back. Nature Neuroscience. 2013;**16**(7):838-844

[14] Edmond EC, Stagg CJ, Turner MR. Therapeutic non-invasive brain stimulation in amyotrophic lateral sclerosis: Rationale, methods and experience. Journal of Neurology, Neurosurgery & Psychiatry. 2019; **90**(10):1131-1138

[15] Wassermann EM, Grafman J. Recharging cognition with DC brain polarization. Trends in Cognitive Sciences. 2005;**9**(11):503-505

[16] Paulus W. Transcranial direct current stimulation (tDCS). In: Supplements to Clinical Neurophysiology. Vol. 56. United States: Elsevier; 2003. pp. 249-254

[17] Kakuda W, Abo M, Kobayashi K, Momosaki R, Yokoi A, Ito H, et al.

Low-frequency rTMS combined with intensive occupational therapy for upper limb hemiparesis after brain tumour resection. Brain Injury. 2010;**24**(12):1505-1510

[18] Khedr EM, Ahmed MA, Fathy N, Rothwell JC. Therapeutic trial of repetitive transcranial magnetic stimulation after acute ischemic stroke. Neurology. 2005;**65**(3):466-468

[19] Darling WG, Wolf SL, Butler AJ. Variability of motor potentials evoked by transcranial magnetic stimulation depends on muscle activation. Experimental Brain Research. 2006; **174**(2):376-385

[20] Loo CK, Taylor JL, Gandevia SC, McDarmont BN, Mitchell PB, Sachdev PS. Transcranial magnetic stimulation (TMS) in controlled treatment studies: Are some "sham" forms active? Biological Psychiatry. 2000;**47**(4):325-331

[21] Opie GM, Liao W-Y, Semmler JG. Interactions between cerebellum and the intracortical excitatory circuits of motor cortex: A mini-review. The Cerebellum. 2021:1-8

[22] Di Pino G, Pellegrino G, Assenza G, Capone F, Ferreri F, Formica D, et al. Modulation of brain plasticity in stroke: A novel model for neurorehabilitation. Nature Reviews Neurology. 2014; **10**(10):597-608

[23] Wolf SL, Winstein CJ, Miller JP, Taub E, Uswatte G, Morris D, et al. Effect of constraint-induced movement therapy on upper extremity function 3 to 9 months after stroke: The EXCITE randomized clinical trial. Journal of the American Medical Association. 2006;**296**(17):2095-2104

[24] Jung SH, Shin JE, Jeong Y-S, Shin H-I. Changes in motor cortical excitability induced by high-frequency repetitive transcranial magnetic stimulation of different stimulation durations. Clinical Neurophysiology. 2008;**119**(1):71-79

[25] Dang G, Chen X, Chen Y, Zhao Y, Ouyang F, Zeng J. Dynamic secondary degeneration in the spinal cord and ventral root after a focal cerebral infarction among hypertensive rats. Scientific Reports. 2016;**6**(1):1-9

[26] Kumru H, Kofler M, Valls-Sole J. Modulation of brainstem reflexes induced by non-invasive brain stimulation: Is there a future? Neural Regeneration Research. 2021;**16**(10):2004

[27] Thut G, Miniussi C. New insights into rhythmic brain activity from TMS–EEG studies. Trends in Cognitive Sciences. 2009;**13**(4):182-189

[28] Groppa S, Oliviero A, Eisen A, Quartarone A, Cohen L, Mall V, et al. A practical guide to diagnostic transcranial magnetic stimulation: Report of an IFCN committee. Clinical Neurophysiology. 2012;**123**(5):858-882

[29] Nair DG, Renga V, Lindenberg R, Zhu L, Schlaug G. Optimizing recovery potential through simultaneous occupational therapy and non-invasive brain-stimulation using tDCS. Restorative Neurology and Neuroscience. 2011;**29**(6):411-420

[30] Boonzaier J, van Tilborg GA, Neggers SF, Dijkhuizen RM. Noninvasive brain stimulation to enhance functional recovery after stroke: Studies in animal models. Neurorehabilitation and Neural Repair. 2018;**32**(11):927-940

[31] Yoon KJ, Lee Y-T, Han TR. Mechanism of functional recovery after repetitive transcranial magnetic stimulation (rTMS) in the subacute cerebral ischemic rat model: Neural plasticity

or anti-apoptosis? Experimental Brain Research. 2011;**214**(4):549-556

[32] Schlaug G, Marchina S, Wan CY. The use of non-invasive brain stimulation techniques to facilitate recovery from post-stroke aphasia. Neuropsychology Review. 2011;**21**(3):288-301

[33] Simonetta-Moreau M. Non-invasive brain stimulation (NIBS) and motor recovery after stroke. Annals of Physical and Rehabilitation Medicine. 2014;**57**(8):530-542

[34] Lindenberg R, Renga V, Zhu L, Nair D, Schlaug G. Bihemispheric brain stimulation facilitates motor recovery in chronic stroke patients. Neurology. 2010;**75**(24):2176-2184

[35] Benjamin EJ, Blaha MJ, Chiuve SE, Cushman M, Das SR, Deo R, et al. Heart disease and stroke statistics—2017 update: A report from the American Heart Association. Circulation. 2017; **135**(10):e146-e603

[36] Hamann G, Bruckmann H. Part C: Functional imaging IN acute stroke, recovery and rehabilitation. This page intentionally left blank. 2002;**96**:48

[37] Pate J, McCambridge A. Single case experimental design: A new approach for non-invasive brain stimulation research? Frontiers in Neuroergonomics. 2021

[38] Narasimhan P, Liu J, Song YS, Massengale JL, Chan PH. VEGF stimulates the ERK 1/2 signaling pathway and apoptosis in cerebral endothelial cells after ischemic conditions. Stroke. 2009;**40**(4):1467-1473

[39] Li W, Li Y, Zhu W, Chen X. Changes in brain functional network connectivity after stroke. Neural Regeneration Research. 2014;**9**(1):51

[40] Stagg CJ, Bachtiar V, O'Shea J, Allman C, Bosnell RA, Kischka U, et al. Cortical activation changes underlying stimulation-induced behavioural gains in chronic stroke. Brain. 2012;**135**(1):276-284

[41] Hordacre B, Moezzi B, Ridding MC. Neuroplasticity and network connectivity of the motor cortex following stroke: A transcranial direct current stimulation study. Human Brain Mapping. 2018;**39**(8):3326-3339

[42] Bashir S, Sikaroudi H, Kazemi R, Forough B, Ekhtiari H. Integrated technologies like noninvasive brain stimulation (NIBS) for stroke rehabilitation new hopes for patients, neuroscientists, and clinicians in Iran. Basic and Clinical Neuroscience. 2010;**1**(4):6-14

[43] Riggall K, Forlini C, Carter A, Hall W, Weier M, Partridge B, et al. Researchers' perspectives on scientific and ethical issues with transcranial direct current stimulation: An international survey. Scientific Reports. 2015;**5**(1):1-10

[44] Rossi S, Hallett M, Rossini PM, Pascual-Leone A, Group SoTC. Safety, ethical considerations, and application guidelines for the use of transcranial magnetic stimulation in clinical practice and research. Clinical Neurophysiology. 2009;**120**(12):2008-2039

[45] Costello A. Repetitive Transcranial Magnetic Stimulation (rTMS) Systems - Class II Special Controls Guidance for Industry and Food and Drug Administration Staff: Class II Special Controls Guidance Document: Repetitive Transcranial Magnetic Stimulation (rTMS) Systems. United States: Food and Drug Administration; 2011

[46] Boes AD, Kelly MS, Trapp NT, Stern AP, Press DZ, Pascual-Leone A.

Noninvasive brain stimulation: Challenges and opportunities for a new clinical specialty. The Journal of Neuropsychiatry and Clinical Neurosciences. 2018;**30**(3):173-179

[47] Lüdemann-Podubecká J, Bösl K, Rothhardt S, Verheyden G, Nowak DA. Transcranial direct current stimulation for motor recovery of upper limb function after stroke. Neuroscience & Biobehavioral Reviews. 2014;**47**:245-259

[48] VanHaerents S, Chang BS, Rotenberg A, Pascual-Leone A, Shafi MM. Noninvasive brain stimulation in epilepsy. Journal of Clinical Neurophysiology. 2020;**37**(2):118-130

Chapter 8

The Cerebral Plasticity Prospect of Stingless Bee Honey-Polyphenols Supplementation in Rehabilitation of Post-Stroke Vascular Cognitive Impairment

Sabarisah Hashim, Che Mohd Nasril Che Mohd Nassir, Mohd Haniff Abu Zarim, Khaidatul Akmar Kamaruzaman, Sanihah Abdul Halim, Mahaneem Mohamed and Muzaimi Mustapha

Abstract

The neuroprotective potential of stingless bee honey (SBH) is still to be documented from numerous studies including that of its effect on cerebrovascular event. This review should guide stroke rehabilitation specialties to a high understanding of the overall circuit changes post-stroke, the clinical relevance of this change in stroke to cognitive impairment and dementia, and SBH as a supplementation in modern stroke rehabilitation in progresses. However, the potential of SBH as a supplementation therapy and highlights treatment to induced plasticity for post-stroke vascular cognitive impairment (PSVCI) remains largely unexplored. This Chapter attempts to deliberate on recent evidence that highlight the therapeutic properties of honey and SBH, the features of PSVCI, and proposing the plausible mechanism of action for SBH as a supplementation during stroke rehabilitation that could halt the progression of PSVCI. It is hoped that such an approach could complement the existing evidence-based stroke care, and which will help in the development of future direction of brain plasticity to delay the progression of cognitive impairment post-stroke.

Keywords: stingless bee honey, plasticity, stroke, post-stroke vascular cognitive impairment, rehabilitation, stroke survivors

1. Introduction

Stroke, whether ischemic or hemorrhage is the phenomena of brain infarction resulted from the alteration of blood supply to the brain tissue leading to cause of death and disabilities. American Heart Association [1] reported that stroke is third leading cause of death and disabilities worldwide, which the global prevalence of stroke in 2019 was 101.5 million people, whereas that ischemic stroke was 77.2 million, that of intracerebral hemorrhage was 20.7 million and that of subarachnoid hemorrhage was 8.4 million [1]. Specific to post-stroke vascular cognitive impairment (PSVCI), it is a syndrome that includes all neurological disorders from mild cognitive impairment to dementia caused by cerebral vascular disease that occurred within three months after stroke onset [2, 3]. PSVCI prevalence is reported between 36 to 67% of survivors and the studies demonstrated that stroke increase risk of persistent and cognitive decline in particular in executive functioning [4–6]. The knowledge pertaining the PSVCI remain in active research, given that a stroke may induce VCI through multiple mechanisms that are often cumulative or synergistic. Thus, a better understanding from the molecular to cellular processes involved in the neuro-gliovascular unit dysfunction may also help to improved prevention and treatments for PSVCI.

Increasing body of evidence had shown that honey exert several medicinal beneficial effects such as gastroprotective [7] reproductive [8, 9] hepatoprotective [10], antihyperglycemic [11] antioxidant [11] and anti-inflammatory [12, 13] properties. SBH or Trigona Honey which is rich in polyphenols is an antioxidant has been shown to prevent neuroinflammation, promote learning, memory, and cognitive function, and protect against neurotoxin-induced neuronal injury in the brain [14–17]. Therefore, this Chapter attempts to describe the cerebral plasticity prospect of SBH - polyphenols supplementation in rehabilitation of PSVCI.

2. Stroke

Stroke is a disease affecting the blood vessel (i.e., arteries) leading to and within the brain. Stroke occurs when a blood vessel that carries oxygen and nutrients to the brain is either blocked by a clot or bursts (or ruptures). When that happens, part of the brain becomes deprived of the blood (and oxygen) it needs, resulting in rapid brain cells death leading to stroke [5]. Stroke is defined as a disruption of blood supply to a part of the brain characteristic by rapid developing of clinical signs of focal (or global) disturbance of cerebral function, resulting in ischemic and tissue death with no apparent cause other than that of vascular origin [18].

2.1 Classification of stroke and location

Stroke has been classified into two major types; firstly, hemorrhagic stroke and secondly is ischemic stroke [1]. The classification of hemorrhagic stroke i.e., due to blood vessel ruptured and bleeding in the brain includes subarachnoid (SAH) and intracerebral hemorrhage (ICH) [1], and for ischemic stroke largely based on the vascular occlusion [19]. The most widely used TOAST classification includes large vessel atherothrombosis (i.e., atherosclerotic disease), cardiogenic embolic or cardio embolism, small artery thrombosis or small vessel disease (i.e., lacunar stroke), other determined causes, and cryptogenic (undetermined causes—include cases involving more than one primary mechanism) [19, 20].

Moreover, stroke is divided into two broad categories according to the lesion location in the brain and vascular territory. Firstly, is anterior (carotid) artery circulation that include middle cerebral artery (MCA) territory, approximately 85% of these are ischemic stroke that mostly led to aphasia (dominant hemisphere), hemiparesis or hemiplegia, hemisensory loss or disturbance, homonymous hemianopia, parietal lobe dysfunction (e.g., astereognosis, agrapha-esthesia, impaired two-point discrimination, sensory and visual inattention, left–right dissociation, and acalculia) [21]. Whilst stroke in anterior cerebral artery (ACA) will lead to weakness of lower limbs more than the upper limbs [22]. Secondly, stroke occur in posterior (or vertebrobasilar) artery circulation, responsible for 20% of all strokes and it feeds the posterior region of the brain, including brainstem, the thalamus, the cerebellum and areas of the occipital and temporal lobes, clinically patient can present with homonymous hemianopia, cortical blindness, ataxia, dizziness or vertigo, dysarthria, diplopia, dysphagia, Horner's syndrome, hemiparesis or hemisensory loss contralateral to the cranial nerves palsy, and cerebellar sign [23].

2.2 Risk factors of stroke

The risk factors for stroke can be classified as modifiable or non-modifiable [17, 24, 25]. Modifiable risk factors that are less specific and more prevalent for example for ischemic stroke the modifiable risk factors includes cardiac disease, diabetes, history of hypertension, hypercholesterolemia, transient ischemic attacks (TIAs), cigarette smoking, hyperhomocysteinemia, obesity, and low physical activity. Meanwhile the modifiable risk factors for hemorrhagic stroke includes the use of anticoagulant, hypertension, heavy drinking, illegal drug use (especially cocaine and crystal meth) and thrombolytic therapy. All this affect health in several ways and provide opportunities to modify risk in large numbers of people [26]. On the other hand, non-modifiable risk factors such as age (stroke risk doubling with each decade of life after the age of 55 years), and race or ethnicity are similar for both ischemic and hemorrhagic stroke. Meanwhile gender (more men have strokes than women; however, more women die of strokes), geographic location, and genetic factors such Fabry's disease may increase risk for ischemic stroke [27].

2.3 Pathophysiology of a stroke

A stroke is a sudden loss of brain function resulting from an interference with the blood supply to the central nervous system (CNS). Normal cerebral blood flow (CBF) is approximately 50–60 ml/100 g/min. The reduction in CBF below 20 ml/100 g/min results in an electrical silence and less than 10 ml/100 g/min causes irreversible neuronal injury [28]. The pathophysiology of stroke is complicated, and associated with excitotoxicity mechanisms, inflammatory pathways, oxidative damage, ionic imbalances, apoptosis, angiogenesis, and neuroprotection. The ultimate result of ischemic cascade initiated by acute stroke is neuronal death along with an irreversible loss of neuronal function [28]. Beside, neuronal cell loss, damage to and loss of astrocytes as well as injury to white matter contributes also to cerebral injury. The core problems in stroke are loss of neuronal cells which makes recovery difficult or even not possible in the late states [29, 30].

Stroke frequently resulting in cerebral edema or secondary ischemia due to mass lesion and subarachnoid hemorrhage, with involvement of hippocampal and frontotemporal regions, causes VCI with visuospatial memory and language deficits [31, 32]. In this case, it is reported that VCI is attributed to the impact of the subdural membrane on dural lymphatic drainage [33]. Therefore, both ischemic and hemorrhagic strokes may lead to a high risk of VCI.

Stroke elicits profound white matter injury, a risk factor for higher stroke incidence and poor neurological outcomes. Depending on the duration and the severity of the ischemic stroke, the effects that are evident in the white matter include activated microglia, clasmatodendritic astrocytosis, and myelin breakdown, presence of axonal bulbs and degeneration and reactivation and loss of oligodendroglia [6]. The majority of damage caused by stroke is located in subcortical regions and, remarkably, white matter occupies nearly half of the average infarct volume [32]. Indeed, white matter is exquisitely vulnerable to ischemia and is often injured more severely than gray matter [32]. The sign and symptoms related to white matter injury include cognitive dysfunction and thus impaired the executive function and verbal fluency, emotional disorders, sensorimotor impairments, as well urinary incontinence and pain, all of this are related to destruction and remodeling of white matter connectivity [32]. A study found that post-stroke survivors who exhibited greater frontal white matter hyperintensities volumes are predicted to have shorter time to dementia onset, with the exhibited disruption of gliovascular interactions and blood brain barrier damage [34]. They also found that, clasmatodendrosis which is linked to white matter hyperintensities, and frontal white matter changes is the substrate that contributed to delayed post- stroke dementia [34].

3. Post stroke vascular cognitive impairment (PSCVI)

Post-stroke cognitive impairment is a new cognitive deficit that begin in first three months following stroke and continue for minimal of six months, which is not explained by any other condition or disease [35]. This deficits occur in 30–40% of individuals in one or more cognitive domains, including language, executive function, visuospatial cognition, episodic and working memory. Moreover, cognitive, affective and behavioral outcome of stroke are more frequently associated with bad quality of life (QoL) than measures of physical disability [35]. While European Stroke Organization (ESO) and European Academy of Neurology (EAN) guideline define post-stroke cognitive impairment as all problems in cognitive function that occur following a stroke, irrespective of the etiology. There is distinction between the broad construct of cognitive impairment and dementia (or major neurocognitive disorder) [36]. However, the risk of dementia after stroke is high, with a post-event incidence of 34% one year after severe stroke (NIHSS>10), with lower rate after TIA and minor stroke [35]. The lesions, such as focal stroke, may disrupt networks either directly, or indirectly, through secondary mechanisms of injury. Specific to neurocognitive impairment post-stroke. **Figure 1** showed a proper account of the consequences of damage to specific areas of brain therefore requires an understanding of the distributed neural networks that underpin these neurocognitive domains and their interaction [35].

3.1 Pathomechanism of PSVCI

Multiple studies had discussed the probable causes of VCI, particularly vascular origin such as reduced blood supply to the brain i.e., cBF [37]. The affected brain areas undergo a neuronal tissue loss which compromises its structure and function and manifests as a VCI. The onset of ischemic cascade showed the initiation of many steps including inflammation, excitotoxicity, nitric oxide production, free radical damage, and apoptosis, all of these play a role in tissue injury. The molecular

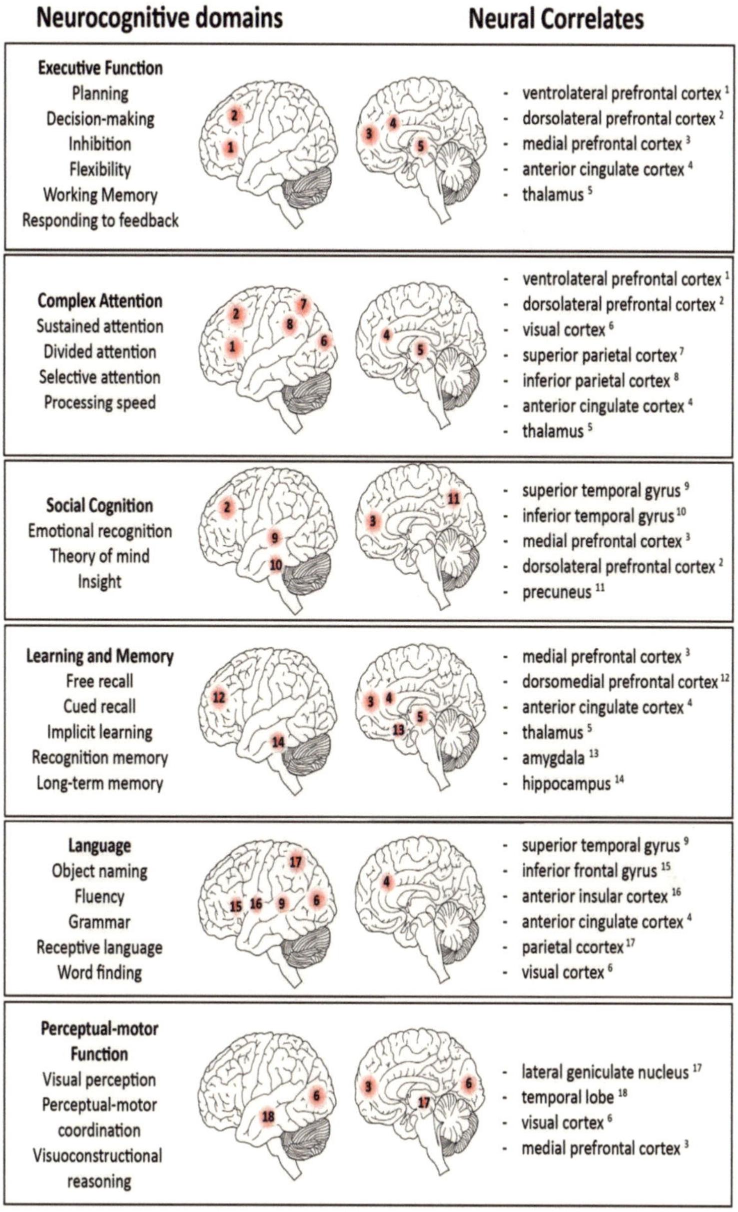

Figure 1.
Neural networks that underpin the neurocognitive domains. Each figure sketches the major regions recognized as part of the network supporting each domain. Key points are that all networks are widely distributed across the brain frequently intersecting and overlapping so that multiple networks may be injured by a single stroke. Copyright from McDonald MW, et al. 2019.

consequences of brain ischemia following a stroke includes temporal change in cell signaling, signal transduction, metabolism, and gene regulation/expression [28, 38].

In the case of stroke, pro-inflammatory mediators, and amyloid deposition (i.e., cerebral amyloid angiopathy [CAA]) in the vessel walls play a crucial role in the development and progression of PSVCI [5, 39]. However, PSVCI generally occurs in a shorter time frame (i.e., less than 1 year) compared to other forms of VCI [40, 41].

The damage caused by CSVD is late onset due to the cortical and subcortical micro-infarcts [42]. The brain region is affected by a state of cerebral hypoperfusion which, in the long term, is responsible for the damage of white matter and for the emergence of cognitive dysfunction [43, 44]. These types of multiple infarctions and diffuse white matter lesions often appear in the lateral ventricle and subcortical structures, resulting in multiple cognitive domain impairments [42–44]. It is also known that VCI can also occur after a cerebral hemorrhage [43, 44], such as CAA-related intracranial hemorrhage [36, 37, 45, 46] that resulting in cerebral edema or secondary ischemia

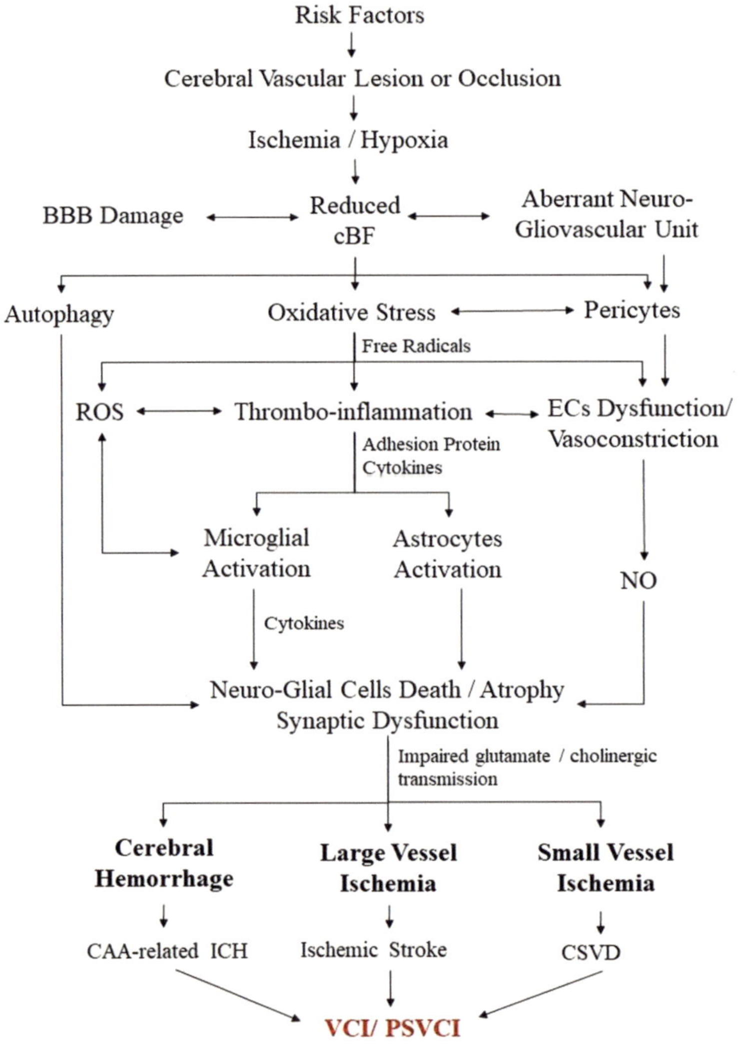

Figure 2.
Proposed general mechanisms on post-stroke vascular cognitive impairment (PSVCI). Crosstalk between the reduced cerebral blood flow (cBF), aberrant neuro-gliovascular unit and blood brain barrier (BBB) damage initiated by ischemic/hypoxic related cerebral vascular lesion and/or occlusion leading to cascade of catastrophic event such as increase reactive oxygen species (ROS), thrombo-inflammation and subsequent endothelial cells dysfunction and/or vasoconstriction. These lead to neuro-glial cells death and synaptic dysfunction, hence cause brain ischemia or hemorrhage and subsequent PSVCI. CAA, cerebral amyloid angiopathy; CSVD, cerebral small vessel disease; ICH, intracerebral hemorrhage; No, nitric oxide; VCI, vascular cognitive impairment.

due to mass lesion and subarachnoid hemorrhage, with involvement of hippocampal and frontotemporal regions, resulting VCI with visuospatial memory and language deficits [38, 39, 47, 48]. In this case, it is reported that VCI is attributed to the impact of the subdural membrane on dural lymphatic drainage [49]. Therefore, both ischemic and hemorrhagic strokes may lead to a high risk of PSVCI.

Figure 2 illustrate the description multiple mechanisms of the PSVCI that include, (1) cerebral vascular lesions (i.e., ischemic or hemorrhages) in a strategic area in terms of cognitive functioning; (2) previous silent CSVD (i.e., leukoaraiosis, cortical microinfarct, silent brain infarcts, cerebral microbleeds, Binswanger leukoencephalopathy, and brain atrophy) that contribute to the burden responsible for VCI through a cumulative effect or dysconnectivity; (3) accelerated evolution of pre-existing degenerative lesions through hypoxia mechanism; (4) direct effect of vascular or metabolic risk factors associated with stroke occurrence on cognitive functioning; (5) direct induction of neurodegeneration responsible for global or regional brain atrophy; (6) endothelial cells dysfunction and blood brain barrier (BBB) damage; and (7) neuro-thrombo-inflammation [6]. A better understanding from the molecular to cellular processes involved in the neuro-gliovascular unit dysfunction may also help to improved prevention and treatments for PSVCI.

Moreover, inflammation and oxidative stress remains an important pathway involved in both neuronal and vascular endothelial dysfunctions [50]. Besides, neurovascular uncoupling is also responsible for disturbance of brain oxygenation and vascular reactivity necessary to supply sufficient cBF in response to neuronal metabolism [51]. In neurohormonal pathways, changes in brain plasticity or neurotrophic factors, ion channels and mitochondrial dysfunction [3, 52, 53] and cognitive dysfunction have all been observed in PSVCI [54]. Interestingly, impairment of neurotransmission pathways, i.e., glutamate or cholinergic transmission has also been associated with cognitive deterioration (**Figure 1**) [55].

Therefore, more clinical, and pre-clinical studies are needed to better characterize all the molecular mechanisms contributing to cellular (i.e., neuronal damage) in PSVCI in order to design for potential pharmacological targets with disease-modifying therapy with pleiotropic compounds or multimodal combinations targeting such as endothelial function and BBB, neuronal death, cerebral plasticity and compensatory mechanism, and degenerative disease-related protein misfolding.

4. Honey and its classification

Honey is the natural sweet substance produced by bees from plants nectar, plant secretions or excretions of plant-sucking insects on the living parts of plants. The bees collect, transform by combining with specific substances of their own, deposit, dehydrate, store, and leave in the honeycomb to ripen and mature [54]. Honey can be classified or categorized according to several properties. Firstly, is bee species, whereby based on the main species of bees, the commercial honey is further categorized as honeybee honey (i.e., produced by all honeybees such as *Apis spp*.) and stingless bee honey (SBH) (i.e., produced by all stingless bees such as *Melipona spp*. and *Trigona spp*.) [55]. Secondly, based on floral or botanical origin or source, whereby honey is also further categorized as unifloral, multifloral, blossom, and) honeydew. The unifloral honey is produced mainly from a single plant species, with identifiable organoleptic characteristics including appearance, color, flavor, and taste, and contains more than 45% of the total pollen from the same plant species as analyzed using visual pollen identification analysis (melissopalynology). The multifloral, also known as polyfloral or blend honey, contains pollen from more than one plant species with no domination by any single plant species [56]. In contrast, the blossom or nectar honey originates from nectars of plants, while honeydew honey comes mainly from excretions of plant sucking insects (Hemiptera) on the living parts of plants or secretions of living parts of plants [54].

Thirdly, it is based on geographical or topographical region of origin, whereby geo- or topographical region is used when honey is exclusively collected and produced within the specific area [57]. Next, is based on the method of beekeeping, where honey is categorized as organic honey which is produced by apiaries with certified organic beekeeping which does not contain toxic residues of pesticides used in agriculture and beekeeping [58]. Besides, honey is also categorized based on the mode of processing, such as squeezed honey when it is obtained by traditionally squeezing the honeycombs, drained honey when it is obtained by draining decapped broodless comb and extracted honey when it is obtained by centrifuging decapped honeycombs which is mainly produced by beekeepers who manage bees in moveable comb hives [58]. The consistency and appearance of honey is also crucial in categorizing the honey for example liquid honey when it is either thinner or thicker in consistency and free of visible crystals, and crystallized honey when it is completely granular or solidified [49].

Moreover, honey can also be classified based on their color, whereby honey color varies from nearly colorless to dark brown [57]. Hence, honey has been categorized as white honey, dark brown or amber and golden honey [49]. However, Department of Agriculture from the United States of America categorizes honey color into seven categories including water white, extra white, white, extra light amber, light amber, amber and dark amber with Pfund color scale of 0 to more than 114 mm [58]. Finally, is based on the style of marketing, honey can be categorized as chunk honey when honey is sold in a piece of a sealed and undamaged honeycomb, comb honey when honey is sold in sealed whole honeycombs, and comb honey in fluid honey when it is sold as a cut honeycomb inserted in fluid honey [56].

5. Stingless bee honey (SBH)

Stingless bee species belonged to the same family as the sting bee, *Hymenoptera*, but classified in a different subfamily level. The stingless bee belongs to the *Meliponinae* subfamily. Like the sting bee, the stingless bee produces honey and other by-products such as bee bread, propolis and royal jelly [59]. Unlike the sting bees, stingless bees store their honey in vertical pots made of cerumen [60]. This part is exclusively known and different to the propolis of the *Apis mellifera*. Propolis, is a natural resinous and waxy product which is produced by mixing beeswax and resins collected from various plant parts. Meanwhile, cerumen is a mixture that similar to propolis but with addition of mandibular secretion of the stingless bee during its construction [61].

Additionally, the stingless bees can be differentiated by the size of their body, which is smaller compared to the sting bees. Apart from being small, the stingless bees have a pot-like structure of honey pot instead of vertical honeycomb produced by the sting bees. There are about 500 species of stingless bees reported with 64 genera distributed in Latin America (*Melipona spp.*, *Tetragonisca spp.*, *Scaptotrigona spp.*, and *Plebeia spp.*), Australia (*Tetragonula spp.*), Africa (*Meliponula spp.*), and

Asia (*Lepidotrigona spp*., *Tetrigona spp*., *Homotrigona* spp., *Lisotrigona* spp.) [62, 63]. In Asia, particularly in Malaysia, more than 30 species of stingless bees from the genus *Trigona spp*. were reported. The most popular species for rearing and having commercial values include *Geniotrigona thoracica* (Smith), *Heterotrigona itama* (Cockerell), *Lepidotrigona terminata* (Smith), *Tetragonula fuscobalteata* (Cameron), and *Tetraponera laeviceps* [64].

SBH, in Malaysia also known as *Kelulut* honey (produced by *Trigona spp*. And *Melipona spp*.) was reported to have distinct features compared to sting bees honey in terms of the taste and the aroma. *Kelulut* honey is stored in clusters of small resin pots that are different from the hexagonal-shaped combs that most are familiar with. It has amber brown appearance and is more diluted as it has high water content compared to the other types of honey. The taste of SBH (i.e., *Kelulut* honey) was reported to be sourer like as well as the aroma, waterier in texture and undergoes a slow crystallization [62].

5.1 Physicochemical composition of SBH

In general, honey contains about 200 distinct compounds [65]. Each honey's composition and properties are uniquely different which depend on the several factors as discussed in Section 3 [55–58]. However, there are many techniques that have been employed to determine the floral and geographical origin of honey produced which include pollen identification, gas chromatography spectrometry, and identification of selected chemical parameters [66].

A good quality honey should have a moisture content that is no more than 20 g/100 g, and a sum of both fructose and glucose that is not less than 60 g/100 g, sucrose content less than 5 g/100 g, free acidity of less than 50 milliequivalents acid per 1 kg (meq/kg), ash content of less than 0.5 g/100 g, diastase activity that is not less than 8 diastase number (DN), hydroxymethylfurfural (HMF) content about less than 40 mg/kg, and electrical conductivity of less than 0.8mS/cm [54, 57]. However, this standard is unfavorable to SBH because it has higher moisture content, invertase activity, and free acidity as well as lower pH and lack of diastase [62, 67]. Therefore, Malaysia Honey production released a standard specifically for Malaysian SBH (MS 2683: 2017) which stated that the quality of raw SBH should follow these requirements: moisture content should be less than 35 g/100 g; sucrose content is less than 7.5 g/100 g, ash content is less than 1.0 g/100 g, HMF content is less than 30 mg/kg, pH between 2.5 to 3.8 and presence of plant phenolics [68].

Apart from geographical origin, the physicochemical properties of honey can also vary depending on the variation of bee species. Although varying, the measured parameters remain common in the SBH compositions, which are the moisture content, followed by free acidity, sugar profile, pH, HMF, ash content, and electrical conductivity. Other frequently studied parameters include enzyme activity, nitrogen, soluble solids, color, minerals, and phenolic compound [69]. **Table 1** summarized the different in physiochemical composition between honey and SBH (based on Malaysia standard) [63, 70–75].

5.2 Minerals and phenolic compound of SBH

Generally, the mineral content of honey is often related to the nutritional benefit of honey [73]. In SBH, a total of 14 minerals are studied and four major minerals are detected in SBH, which are potassium (K^+), Sodium (Na^+), Calcium (Ca^{2+}) and

Composition	Honey	SBH
Moisture	≤ 20 g/100 g	≤ 35 g/100 g
Sugar (i.e., Fructose + Glucose)	≥ 60 g/100 g	≥ 40 g/100 g
Sucrose	< 5 g/100 g	< 7.5 g/100 g
Free Acid	< 50 mg/kg	≤ 50 mg/kg
Ash content	< 0.5 g/100 g	< 1.0 g/100 g
Diastase number (DN)	≥ 8 DN	≥ 5 DN
Hydroxymethylfurfural (HMF) content	< 40 mg/kg	< 30 mg/kg
Electrical conductivity (EC)	0.8 mS/cm	0.1 mS/cm
pH	3.2–4.5	3.15–6.64
Nitrogen content	5–200 mg/kg	107–816 mg/kg

DN, diastase number; EC, electrical conductivity; HMF, Hydroxymethylfurfura; SBH, stingless bee honey; g, gram; mg, milligram, cm; centimeter.

Table 1.
Different in physiochemical composition between honey and SBH (based on Malaysia standard).

Magnesium (Mg^{2+}). The most abundant mineral detected in SBH is K^+, followed by Na^+, Ca^{2+}, and lastly, Mg^{2+} [62, 76].

Moreover, SBH has been reported to have a higher content of polyphenol than any other kind of honey [62]. Therefore, the best indicator for SBH quality is the presence of the plant phenolic compounds. These includes benzoic acid, phenylpropanoic acid, 4-hydroxybenzoic acid, 4-hydroxyphenylacetic acid, vanilic acid, protocatechuic acid and p-coumaric acid [68]. Other phenolic compound reported to be present in SBH are luteolin, gallic acid, salicylic acid, syringic acid, cinnamic acid, naringenin, quercetin, isorhamnetin, apigenin, kaempferol, methyl quercetin, taxifolin, isorhamnetin deoxyhexosyl hexoside, quercetin deoxyhexosyl hexoside, and kaempferol deoxyhexosyl hexoside [75, 76].

5.3 SBH: Health benefits and mechanistic profiles

Modern science has found that most traditional practice of using SBH as a great potential as an added value in modern medicine and considered to have a higher medicinal value than other bee species. As discussed, SBH mays serve as anti-inflammatory, anti-cancer [72] anti-bacterial [77], antioxidant, and anti-tumor [63]. According to several physicochemical criteria, the composition of stingless bee honey differs from that of other species [78].

Moreover, SBH was generously studied and reported to possess varieties health-beneficial effect. A study reported that administration of SBH on male diabetic rats showed an ameliorative effect on the testicular structure and function [79]. Furthermore, SBH also showed a potential as antihyperglycemic agent after being administered for 14 days in diabetic rats [9]. Another study on SBH also reported that SBH showed an antimicrobial activity through an in vitro study [80, 81]. Administration of this honey also reported to increase sperm production and elevate testosterone level in diabetic rats [9]. Traditionally, SBH is used for anti-aging, enhancing libido, treatment for bronchial phlegm, relieving sore throat cough and cold, and improving immune system [82]. Interestingly, *Kelulut* honey has been found to have

Phenolic compounds	Neuroprotective potentials		Cerebral plasticity prospect
	Antioxidants	**Anti-Inflammatory**	
Chrysin	Reduced neuronal damage by decreasing oxidative injury [96].	Against neuronal damage by inhibiting inflammatory response [96].	Protect against memory impairment due to neurodegeneration and ameliorate cognitive deficit [96, 97].
Gallic acid	Promotes cerebral antioxidant defense and excellent free radical scavenger [98]. Reduce oxidative stress cause by 6-OHDA and protect against cognitive impairment [99].	Potent anti-inflammatory agent against vascular disease [100].	Reinstated the spatial memory in animal models of vascular dementia due to the ischemic brain injury [101]. Against the acute and chronic oxidative stress that is the basis of neurodegeneration [102]
Cinnamic acid	Potent oxidative stress reduction capacity and antigenotoxic capacity of *p*-coumaric acid [103].	*p*-Coumaric acid exhibited neuroprotective effects against 5-S-cysteinyl-dopamine-induced neurotoxicity [104].	*p*-Coumaric acid had the potential to be the main element for the prevention or treatment of AD and the development of novel monoamine oxidase inhibitors [105].
Quercetin	Protect against oxidative damage caused by induced cerebral stroke in young and old rats [106]. Attenuated oxidative stress induced by high fat diet in mice and improving spatial learning and memory [107].	Helps in ICH by deterring inflammatory response and apoptosis and reducing lesion volume hence stimulating restoration of neural function [4].	Ameliorate the ischemic injury by regulating acid-sensing ion channel led calcium and lipid peroxidation in neural cell [108]. Enhancing the neuronal count in the hippocampus area, which is the worst affected region post-stroke [109]. Delaying the development of AD and cognitive function deficit [110, 111].
Catechins	Ameliorate oxidative stress-caused by neurodegeneration diseases [112]. Mitigate oxidative stress following the insult caused by the cerebral ischemia [113]. Able to indirectly enhance the body's endogenous antioxidants to fight against the oxidative damage cause by various reasons [113].	Mitigate the inflammatory reaction following the insult caused by the cerebral ischemia [113].	Significant neuroprotective effect against neuronal insult caused by transient global ischemia [114]. High dose may help in attenuating the formation of post-ischemic brain oedema and reduced the volume infarction following the unilateral cerebral ischemia [115]. Improve learning and memory function in aged mice [116].
Apigenin	Protects neurons against oxygen–glucose deprivation/reperfusion-induced injury in cultured primary hippocampal neurons by improving sodium/potassium-ATPase (Na^+/K^+-ATPase) activities [117].	Inhibits the kainic acid-induced excitotoxicity of hippocampal cells in a dose-dependent manner by quenching ROS and by inhibiting the depletion of reduced glutathione levels [118].	Neuroprotective effect against ischemia/reperfusion injury by promoting cell proliferation, reduced cerebral infarct areas, alleviated apoptosis, and improved neurological function [119, 120] Stimulates the adult neurogenesis that underlies learning and memory [93].

Phenolic compounds	Neuroprotective potentials		Cerebral plasticity prospect
	Antioxidants	**Anti-Inflammatory**	
Caffeic Acid	Potent antioxidant against ischemic/ reperfusion injury [121].	Reduce infarct volume and neuroinflammation activity [122].	Neuroprotective effect against ischemic/reperfusion injury and adverse drug reactions [121].
Kaempferol	Ameliorated antioxidant defenses and antiapoptotic effects involve the enhancement of mitochondrial turnover, which is mediated by autophagy [123].	Attenuate ischemic brain damage and inflammation by preventing the activation of STAT3 and NF-κB pathway and ameliorate neurological deficit caused by the ischemic stroke [124].	Administration of kaempferol to ischemic stroke rats' model for 7 days post cerebral ischemia/reperfusion was able to significantly reduce cerebral infarct volume, decreased inflammation and help promoting intact BBB [125]. Optimal treatment for improving cognitive function due to its positive effects on depression, mood, and cognitive functions [126].

6-OHDA, 6-hydroxy dopamine; AD, Alzheimer's disease; ATPase, adenosine triphosphatase; BBB, blood brain barriers; GSH, glutathione; ICH, intracerebral hemorrhages; NF-κB, nuclear factor kappa B; ROS, reactive oxygen species; STAT3, signal transducer and activator of transcription 3.

Table 2.
List of important polyphenols components found in SBH and its neuroprotective potentials (i.e., antioxidants, anti-inflammatory) and their cerebral plasticity prospect.

multitude pharmacological properties, which include anti-inflammatory [83, 84] antibacterial [85, 86], anticancer [86–88] and antioxidant [89, 90].

However, antioxidants (i.e., molecules that slow or stop other molecules from oxidizing) preventing diseases like neurological disorders. Antioxidants protect cell structure by neutralizing ROS and thereby terminating the harmful chain reaction in the body [22]. As discussed, the principal beneficial compounds found in SBH are polyphenols. Polyphenols and phenolic acids are thought to be richer in SBH than in any other type of honey [62, 76]. SBH samples have a much higher antioxidant capacity than *Tualang* honey samples, with statistically significant relationships between antioxidant outcomes and polyphenols concentration ($p < 0.0.05$) interestingly, SBH composition with strong antioxidant and anti-inflammatory factors had been shown to improve cognitive deficits [8, 9], namely from high flavonoids and polyphenols that protect against neurodegenerative disorders through modulating neuronal and glial signaling pathways (10).

High polyphenols content in SBH (i.e., *Kelulut* honey) can help to ameliorate PSVCI due to the oxidative damage thus providing an inexpensive neuroprotective therapeutic role. Not only dietary polyphenols can help in protecting brain from oxidative-stress injury, it also can mitigate neuroinflammation [91] protecting against neurodegeneration and promoting learning and memory and cognitive function [71, 92, 93]. Additionally, polyphenols are the significant bioactive molecules which act as the antioxidant that present in honey that may contribute relatively to the proven pharmacological properties of the SBH (i.e., *Kelulut* honey) [94]. *Kelulut* honey has been proven to have higher content of polyphenol than other honey [76, 84]. There is significant correlation between high polyphenol content to the antioxidant properties [76]. The common groups of polyphenols that have been detected are flavonoids and phenolic acid. There are several most reported phenolic and flavonoid compounds that can be found in *Kelulut* honey which may help in alleviating or reversing the cognitive decline in post-stroke patients, namely gallic acid, caffeic acid, catechin, apigenin, chrysin, cinnamic acid, kaempferol, p-coumaric acid and quercetin [78, 95]. Several important polyphenols components that can be found in *Kelulut* honey and act as neuroprotective (i.e., antioxidants and anti-inflammatory) and aided in cerebral plasticity following PSVCI is summarized in **Table 2**.

6. Cerebral plasticity prospect of SBH supplementation in rehabilitation of PSVCI

Cerebral plasticity of SBH supplementation in rehabilitation for PSVCI have been developed with two main aims: restoration of cerebral flow and the minimization of the deleterious effects of ischemia on neurons, [28] and the mechanism of polyphenols in SBH as neuroprotective in brain reported able to prevent neuro-inflammation, promote memory, learning and cognitive function and protect against neurotoxin-induced neuronal injury, hence improved the defend mechanism against oxidative stress, neuro-inflammation and attenuated free radical-mediated molecular destruction [14, 92]. There are ongoing studies to investigate the potential positive effect of flavonoids from honey as cerebral plasticity prospect to delay the progression of cognitive impairment [17].

6.1 Prevent neuro-inflammation

Inflammation has been identified as important factor in the pathogenic mechanisms of cerebrovascular disease and neurodegenerative disease such as dementia [127]. There are evidence that chronic inflammation involved in the pathogenesis of several condition post-stroke and dementia. Human and animal studies indicates that inflammation mediated by inflammatory cells, cytokines, cell adhesion molecules, and eicosanoids occurs after ischemic injury and may exacerbate ischemic injury [28]. The mechanism in vascular damage seen in brain is encourage and maintain by cytokines, acute phase proteins, endothelial cell adhesive molecular and other immune-related protein. Microvascular inflammation is a hypo-perfusion model with markers of chronic inflammation and endothelial activation, can lead to increase BBB permeability and to infiltration of inflammatory factors like interleukins, MMPs, Tumor necrosis factors (TNFα), toll like receptor 4 (TLR4) and C-reaction protein (CRP). This product upon enter into brain, these inflammatory factors can exacerbate white matter damage [127], in early in the pathology process of Alzheimer disease in patients with mild cognitive impairment (MCI) [128].

Human and animal studies indicates that inflammation mediated by inflammatory cells, cytokines, the cell adhesion molecules, and eicosanoids occurs after ischemic injury and may exacerbate ischemic injury [28]. The common studies biomarkers in VCI and dementia are interleukin-6 (IL-6), MMPs, Tumor necrosis factors (TNFα), toll like receptor 4 (TLR4) and C-reactive protein (CRP) [17].

Potential therapeutic targets to minimize tissue loss and neurologic deficit by lessening the proportion of penumbral tissue recruited into the infection area. Inflammation occurs by molecular and cellular components at blood-microvacular endothelial cell interface [28]. SBH with phenolic acid consumption is an antioxidant that act as neuroprotective effect to prevent neuro-inflammation, promote memory, learning, cognitive function and protect against neurotoxin-induced neuronal injury in brain [14, 16, 129]. Flavonoid or myricetin modulates an interleukin −1 beta − mediated inflammatory response in human astrocytes in alleviation of neuroinflammation [15].

In this perspective, the role of honey as one of the natural supplements worth to be explored for its potential in halting the progression of cognitive impairment and dementia [15, 16, 95]. Nevertheless, to our best knowledge, limited such study exists on stroke patients whether with cognitive or physical impairment with the used of honey in promoting recovery in functional and to delay the progression of impairments.

6.2 Against oxidative stress

As mentioned earlier in this chapter, oxidative stress in brain tissue had been proven to contribute to reducing cognitive function in aging brain [130]. Oxidative stress defines the inadequate balance between free radicals and antioxidant protective activity [129]. Oxidate stress is a common manifestation of all type of biochemical insults to the structural and functional integrity of neural cells, such as aging, neuroinflammation, development of neurological disease (Alzheimer disease and Parkinson's disease) and neurotoxins [14, 16]. In addition, increased oxidative stress may impair learning [78] and memory [131] thus overall cognitive function. It has been proven also that oxidative stress is part of the pathology of traumatic brain injury (TBI) and impairs the neuronal function [129]. Oxidative stress biomarkers had been found to be increased within 24-hour post onset of acute ischemic stroke and reduced within 3 months due to the activated antioxidant system [132]. Taking all together, this prove that oxidative stress plays a part in reducing cognitive function post-stroke that impair learning and memory.

Honey with an antioxidant property such as phenolic acid can decrease oxidative stress by improved the defend mechanism against oxidative stress and attenuated free radical-mediated molecular destruction [14–16, 129]. One of SBH most essential characteristics is their antioxidant ability, which helps to prevent certain diseases by protecting cells from oxidative agents like free radicals.

6.3 Increase learning and memory

The progression of cognitive impairment or dementia post stroke can be delayed or prevented by introducing honey as supplementary therapy in early stage of stroke patient with mild cognitive impairment in animal study [9, 92, 93, 133]. Honey was reported can against chronic cerebral hypoperfusion such as in Alzheimer's disease and effect on memory and learning process such as in prevent dementia. Studied the use of honey as a natural preventive therapy of cognitive decline and dementia in 2893 subjects in Iraq. Only 95 from 1495 subject who received honey were found to develop dementia (6.35%) as compared to placebo group (n = 1400) whereby 394 subjects developed dementia (28.1%) ($p < 0.05$) [15]. This study suggested that honey and its properties act as natural preventive therapies for both cognitive impairment and dementia but still less evidence to support the association between honey and the progression of dementia. Concerning neurodegenerative disorder, honey (*Tualang*) was found to have significant activity against chronic cerebral hypoperfusion that have protective effects in learning and memory, which is one of several factors contributing to dementia and Alzheimer's disease (AD) [76].

Honey also showed able to enhance memory by effect to increase proliferation of neuron in hippocampal region [16, 93]. Study reported that reported that both short and long term and supplementations with honey at a dose of 230 mg/kg of body weight significantly decreased the number of degenerated neuronal cells in hippocampus region, which acts as defense mechanism against stress [93].

The study finding stated that SBH supplementation effect and increase learning and memory performance of brain and it is because content of high antioxidant that enhance synaptic plasticity through synaptogenesis in brain [92]. It is because quercetin is another flavonoid with antioxidant activity found in honey improves memory and hippocampal synaptic plasticity in models of memory impairment that cause by chronic lead exposure. Quercetin also has neuroprotective effect against colchicine-induced cognitive impairment [95]. While Cafeic acid present in honey give an effect as neuroprotective on neuronal cell in brain in prevention learning and memory deficit and catechin contribute as antioxidant that give effect as neuroprotection on neuronal cell that delay memory impairment. Finding of studies reported that honey is significantly reduced molecular destruction and improvement in the memory performance that delay the progression of cognitive impairment or dementia [133].

Recent study showed that one of the components of SBH from *Trigona* spp. (i.e., phenylalanine) may be able to trigger the upregulation of brain-derived neurotrophic factor (BDNF) and inositol 1, 4, 5-triphosphate receptor type 1 (ITPR1) [95, 134] which are genes involved in synaptic function [135]. Therefore, trigona displayed capabilities in improving cerebral plasticity (especially after PSVCI) including spatial working memory, spatial reference memory and memory consolidations. Another study also suggested that SBH improves memory and reduces anxiety, in addition to its potential to reduce triglyceride, LDL, and normalize blood glucose in rats with metabolic syndrome [94].

6.4 Attenuated free radical-mediated molecular destruction

Free radical lead to protein dysfunction, DNA damage, and lipid peroxidation, resulting in cell death due to the disruption of the blood–brain barrier in stroke. Free radicals are highly unstable, and therefore very reactive atoms, molecules, or compounds due to their atomic or molecular structure, which has one or more unpaired electrons. They attempt to pair up with other molecules, atoms, or even individual's electrons to create a stable compound, receiving electrons from other atoms [131]. This generates reactive oxygen species (ROS) and free radicals that can bring about molecular transformation and gene mutations in many types of organisms. This is called oxidative stress and is deemed to contribute to the development of chronic and neurodegenerative diseases such as Alzheimer disease that could lead to dementia [12]. ROS are produced naturally by metabolism such as due to the inflammation or result from poor living conditions and environmental pollution. The radical theory in human physiology claims that active free radicals are involved in almost all cellular degradation processes and lead to cell death.

In order to better clinical prognosis, more studies focus on pharmaceutical and non-pharmaceutical neuroprotective therapies against free radical damage [136]. Honey with high phenolic acid can improved the defend mechanism against attenuated free radical-mediated molecular destruction [14, 15]. As reported, apigenin in honey provide as radical scavenging activity where it is protects neuron against oxygen–glucose deprivation/reperfusion-induced injury in cultured primary hippocampal neuross by improving sodium/potassium ATPase ($Na+/K+$ -ATPase) activities [15].

6.5 Polyphenols as anti-acetylcholinesterase activity

Loss of cholinergic activity, atrophy of the nucleus basalts of Meynert as the major source of acetylcholine (Ach), and loss of cortically projecting cholinergic neurons, as well as increased cognitive deficits, are some of the notable findings in various neurodegenerative diseases such as AD, Parkinson disease, and dementia

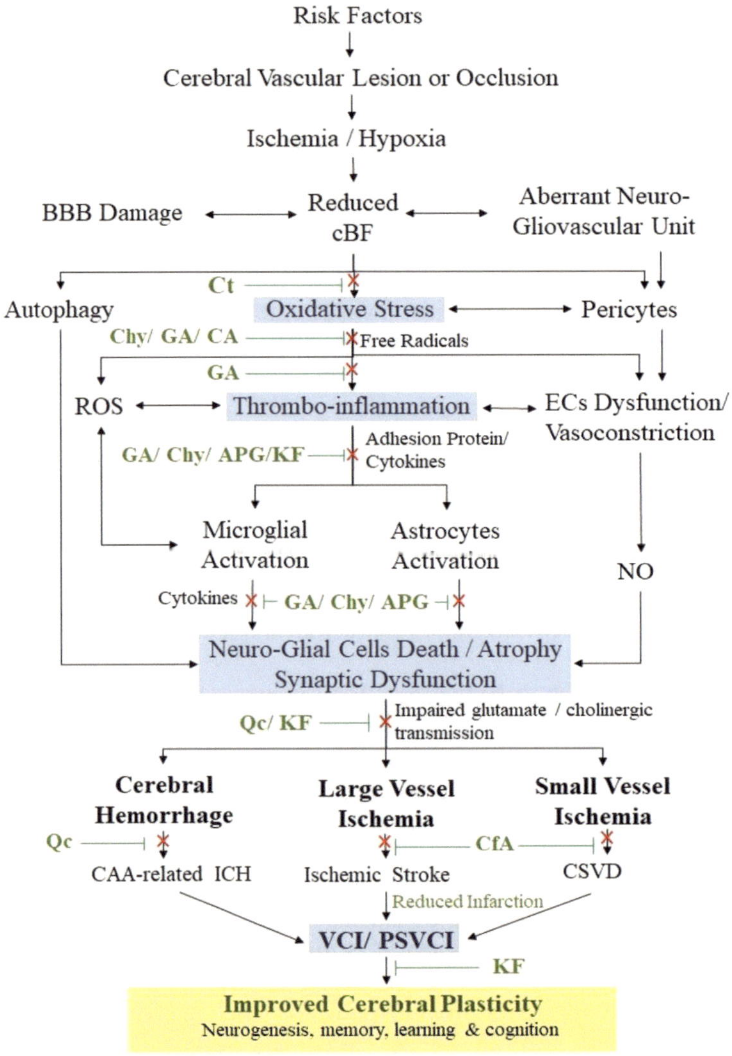

Figure 3.
The proposed mechanism of action of SBH derived polyphenols. Catechins (Ct) enhance the body's endogenous antioxidants to fight against the oxidative stress. Chrysin (Chy), gallic acid (GA), and cinnamic acid (CA) are potent antioxidants, and radical scavengers, hence protect against oxidative damage. GA also potent anti-thrombo-inflammatory agent. Apigenin (APG), kaempferol (KF), GA, and Chy ameliorated antioxidant defenses and reduced thrombo-inflammatory reaction, hence attenuate neuro-glial cells death, atrophy and reduced synaptic dysfunction. Quercetin (Qc) and KF also serve as anti-cholinesterase activity and improve cholinergic transmission. Caffeic acid (CfA) is a potent antioxidant against ischemia and help reduce neuroinflammation and infarct volume. Optimal treatment of SBH-derived polyphenols may improve cerebral plasticity following post-stroke vascular cognitive impairment (PSVCI) – in term of neurogenesis, memory, learning and cognition.

and including PSVCI. Diminished Ach synthesis owing to reduced choline acetyltransferase, choline absorption, cholinergic neuronal and axonal abnormalities, and cholinergic neuron death can all cause cholinergic dysfunction in neurodegenerative disorders [137].

As a result, utilizing acetylcholinesterase inhibitors, which work by stimulating both the muscarinic and nicotinic acetylcholine receptors, has proven to be an effective treatment for the cognitive symptoms of neurodegenerative disease [138]. In the brain, there are two different types of Ach receptors: ligand gated nicotinic Ach receptors (nAChRs) and metabotropic muscarinic Ach receptors (mAChRs). mAChRs are divided into five subtypes (M1-M5). The most prevalent subtype of M1 mAChR is found in the cerebral cortex and hippocampus, which are the most vulnerable brain areas to the formation of amyloid plaques and neurofibrillary tangles [139]. Some polyphenols found in SBH have been proven to inhibit cholinesterase. The anti-cholinergic effect of polyphenol was accompanied by improvements in cognitive function, such as learning and memory, in most *in vivo* investigations [140]. In a study, resveratrol was found to inhibit acetylcholine release from adrenal chromaffin cells. Huperzine A, Quercetin, Kuwanon U, E, and C, kaempferol, tri- and tetrahydroxyflavone, and other polyphenols found in SBH have an anti-butyrylcholinesterase activity in addition to anti-cholinesterase activity [140].

Huperzine A of polyphenols has the highest acetylcholinesterase (AChE) inhibitory activity after donepezil, while tacrine, physostigmine, galantamine, and rivastigmine were less potent. Huperzine A has also shown better penetration through the.

BBB, higher oral bioavailability, and longer duration of Ache-l activity [140]. Clinical trials with Huperzine A, for treatment of cognitive and functional impairments of AD and schizophrenia and the increase in memory performance of normal individuals, have been promising [141, 142]. In China, Huperzine A has been studied in phase IV clinical trials and revealed a significant improvement of memory of elderly people, patients with AD and patients with vascular dementia [138]. Several meta-analyses have shown that administration of Huperzine A for at least 8 weeks might lead to a significant improvement in cognitive function, mood, behavior, and daily activity of patients with AD [142, 143].

Taking all together, polyphenol compounds that can be found in SBH have the neuroprotective effect to ameliorate many neurological deficits and any improve cerebral plasticity during neurorehabilitation after PSVCI. This shows the huge potential of SBH (i.e., *Kelulut* honey) to become a therapeutic treatment and neurorehabilitation in stroke and PSVCI. The proposed mechanism of action of SBH derived polyphenols is described in **Figure 3**.

7. Conclusions

In this chapter, we highlighted the neuroprotective potential and cerebral plasticity prospect of SBH as a dietary supplementation, specifically for PSVCI. Further translational and clinical research can consider the putative mechanisms of action as deliberated here to demonstrate its beneficial impact it may have on cerebral plasticity as part of stroke rehabilitation. It is hoped that such an approach could complement the existing evidence-based stroke care and contribute to halt the progression of vascular cognitive impairment among stroke survivors.

Acknowledgements

The authors express their gratitude to the Universiti Sains Malaysia, especially the Research University Individual (RUI)-Special Grant Scheme with project No: 1001/PPSP/8012384, Project Code: UO2026 (Reference No: 2021/0310) and Universiti Sains Malaysia, Short Term Grant (STG) 2020 with project No:304/PPSP/6315445, that have been granted for Stingless Bee Honey RCT project and, more specifically in exploring the prospect of stingless bee honey (SBH) as the neuroprotective intervention in stroke rehabilitation against vascular cognitive impairment (VCI).

Conflict of interest

The authors declare no conflict of interest.

Notes/thanks/other declarations

Thanks for all.

Author details

Sabarisah Hashim[1,2*†], Che Mohd Nasril Che Mohd Nassir[1†], Mohd Haniff Abu Zarim[2,3], Khaidatul Akmar Kamaruzaman[4], Sanihah Abdul Halim[2,3], Mahaneem Mohamed[2,4] and Muzaimi Mustapha[1,2]

1 Department of Neurosciences, School of Medical Sciences, Universiti Sains Malaysia, Kubang Kerian, Kelantan, Malaysia

2 Hospital Universiti Sains Malaysia, Kubang Kerian, Kelantan, Malaysia

3 Department of Internal Medicine, School of Medical Sciences, Universiti Sains Malaysia, Kubang Kerian, Kelantan, Malaysia

4 Department of Physiology, School of Medical Sciences, Universiti Sains Malaysia, Kubang Kerian, Kelantan, Malaysia

*Address all correspondence to: risha@usm.my

† Co-first author.

References

[1] https://www.heart.org//2021-Heart-and-Stroke. StatUpdate/2021_Stat_Update_factsheet_Global_Burden_of_Disease.pdf

[2] Bordet R, Ihl R, Korczyn AD, et al. Towards the concept of disease- modifier in post-stroke or vascular cognitive impairment: A consensus report. BMC Medicine. 2017, 2016;**15**(1):107-107

[3] Mijajlović MD et al. Post-stroke dementia: A comprehensive review. BMC Medicine. 2017;**15**:1-12

[4] Zhang Y, Yi B, Ma J, Zhang L, Zhang H, Yang Y, et al. Quercetin promotes neuronal and behavioral recovery by suppressing inflammatory response and apoptosis in a rat model of intracerebral hemorrhage. Neurochemical Research. 2015;**40**(1): 195-203

[5] Caplan LR. Basic pathology, anatomy, and pathophysiology of stroke. In: Caplan's Stroke: A Clinical Approach. 4th ed. Philadelphia: Saunders Elsevier; 2009. p. 22

[6] Kalaria RN. Vascular basis for brain degeneration: Faltering controls and risk factors for dementia. Nutrition Reviews. 2010;**68**(suppl_2):S74-S87. DOI: 10.1111/j.1753-4887.2010.00352.x

[7] Gharzouli K, Amira S, Gharzouli A, Khennouf S. Gastroprotective effects of honey and glucose-fructose-sucrose-maltose mixture against ethanol-, indomethacin- and acidified aspirin-induced lesions in the rat. Experimental and Toxicologic Pathology. 2002;**54**:217-221

[8] Mohamed M, Sulaiman SA, Jaafar H, Sirajudeen KN. Effect of different doses of Malaysian honey on reproductive parameters in adult male rats. Andrologia. 2012;**44**(S1):182-186

[9] Kamaruzzaman MA, Chin KY, Mohd Ramli ES. A review of potential beneficial effects of honey on bone health. Evidence-based Complementary and Alternative Medicine. 2019:8543618. DOI: 10.1155/2019/8543618

[10] Al-Waili NS, Saloom KY, Al-Waili TN, Al-Waili AN, Akmal M, Al-Waili FS, et al. Influence of various diet regimens on deterioration of hepatic function and hematological parameters following carbon tetrachloride: A potential protective role of natural honey. Natural Product Research. 2006;**20**:1258-1264

[11] Erejuwa OO, Gurtu S, Sulaiman SA, Ab Wahab MS, Sirajudeen KN, Salleh MS. Hypoglycemic and antioxidant effects of honey supplementation in streptozotocin-induced diabetic rats. International Journal for Vitamin and Nutrition Research. 2010;**80**:74-82

[12] Tan HT, Rahman RA, Gan SH, Halim AS, Hassan SA, Sulaiman SA, et al. The antibacterial properties of Malaysian Tualang honey against wound and enteric microorganisms in comparison to Manuka honey. BMC Complementary and Alternative Medicine. 2009;**9**:34

[13] Kassim M, Achoui M, Mustafa MR, Mohd MA, Yusoff KM. Ellagic acid, phenolic acids and flavonoids in Malaysian honey extracts demonstrate in vitro anti-inflammatory activity. Nutrition Research. 2010;**30**:650-659

[14] Yaacob M, Rajab N, Shahar S, Sharif R. Stingless bee honey and it's potential value: A systematic review. Food Research. 2018

[15] Al-himyari F. The use of honey as a natural preventive therapy of cognitive decline and dementia in the Middle East. Alzheimers & Dementia. 2009:**5**. DOI: 10.1016/j.jalz.2009.04.248

[16] Rao PV, Krishnan KT, Salleh N, Gan SH. Biological and therapeutic effects of honey produced by honey bees and stingless bees: A comparative review. Revista Brasileira de Farmacognosia. 2016;**26**:657-664

[17] Hashim S, Suhana A, Mohammad A, Zulkifli M, Mahaneem M, Rohimah M, et al. Trigona honey as a potential supplementary therapy to halt the progression of post-stroke vascular cognitive impairment. International. International Medical Journal. 1994;**28**(3):335-338

[18] Sacco RL, Benjamin EJ, Broderick JP, et al. American Heart Association Prevention Conference. IV. Prevention and rehabilitation of stroke. Stroke. 1997;**28**(7):1507-1517. DOI: 10.1161/01.STR.28.7.1507

[19] Adams HP Jr, Bendixen BH, Kappelle LJ, et al. Classification of subtype of acute ischemic stroke. Definitions for use in a multicenter clinical trial. TOAST. Trial of Org 10172 in Acute Stroke Treatment. Stroke. 1993;**24**:35-41. DOI: 10.1161/01.STR.24.1.35

[20] Rovira A, GrivÃ E, Rovira A, Alvarez-Sabin J. Distribution territories and causative mechanisms of ischemic stroke. European Radiology. 2005;**15**(3):416-426. DOI: 10.1007/s00330-004-2633-5

[21] Nogles TE, Galuska MA. Middle Cerebral Artery Stroke StatPearls. Treasure Island (FL): StatPearls Publishing Copyright; 2021

[22] Matos Casano HA, Tadi P, Ciofoaia GA. Anterior Cerebral Artery Stroke *StatPearls*. Treasure Island (FL): StatPearls Publishing Copyright; 2021

[23] Nouh A, Remke J, Ruland S. Ischemic posterior circulation stroke: A review of anatomy, clinical presentations, diagnosis, and current management. Frontiers in Neurology. 2014;**5**:30. DOI: 10.3389/fneur.2014.00030

[24] Bamford J, Sandercock P, Dennis M, Burn J, Warlow C. Classification and natural history of clinically identifiable subtypes of cerebral infarction. Lancet. 1991;**337**(8756):1521-1526. DOI: 10.1016/0140-6736(91)93206-o

[25] Allen CL, Bayraktutan U. Risk factors for Ischaemic stroke. International Journal of Stroke. 2008;**3**:105-116

[26] Whisnant JP. Modeling of risk factors for ischemic stroke. Stroke. 1997;**28**(9):1840-1844. DOI: 10.1161/01.str.28.9.1840

[27] Wolf PA, D'Agostino RB, O'Neal MA, et al. Secular trends in stroke incidence and mortality: The Framingham Study. Stroke. 1992;**23**:1551-1555. DOI: 10.1161/01.STR.23.11.1551

[28] Mir M, Albaradie R, Alhassanavi M. Pathophysiology of Strokes. 2014. pp. 25-80

[29] Sekerdag E, Solaroglu I, Gursoy-Ozdemir Y. Cell death mechanisms in stroke and novel molecular and cellular treatment options. Current Neuropharmacology. 2018;**16**(9):1396-1415

[30] Dichgans M, Leys D. Vascular cognitive impairment. Circulation Research. 2017;**120**(3):573-591. DOI: 10.1161/circresaha.116.308426

[31] Chen S, Shao L, Ma L. Cerebral edema formation after stroke: Emphasis on blood- brain barrier and the lymphatic drainage system of the brain. Frontiers in Cellular Neuroscience. 2021;**15**:716825

[32] Wang Y, Liu G, Hong D, Chen F, Ji X, Cao G. White matter injury in ischemic stroke. gProNeurobiol. 2016;**141**:45-60

[33] Sahyouni R, Goshtasbi K, Mahmoodi A, Tran DK, Chen JW. Chronic subdural hematoma: A perspective on subdural membranes and dementia. World Neurosurgery. 2017;**108**:954-958. DOI: 10.1016/j.wneu.2017.09.063

[34] Chen A, Akinyemi RO, Hase Y, Firbank MJ, Ndung'u MN, Foster V, et al. Frontal white matter hyperintensities, clasmatodendrosis and gliovascular abnormalities in ageing and post-stroke dementia. Brain: A Journal of Neurology. 2016;**139**(Pt 1):242-285

[35] McDonald MW, Black SE, Copland DA, Corbett D, Dijkhuizen RM, Farr TD. et al, Cognition in stroke rehabilitation and recovery research: Consensus-based core recommendations from the second Stroke Recovery and Rehabilitation Roundtable. International Journal of Stroke. 2019;**14**(8):774-782

[36] Quinn TJ, Richard E, Teuschl Y, Gattringer T, Hafdi M, O'Brien JT, et al. European Stroke Organisation and European Academy of Neurology joint guidelines on post-stroke cognitive impairment. European Journal of Neurology. 2021;**28**(12):3883-3920. DOI: 10.1111/ene.15068

[37] Barbay M, Taillia H, Nedelec-Ciceri C, Arnoux, A, Puy L, Wiener E, Roussel M. Vascular cognitive impairment: Advances and trends. Revue Neurologique, 2017;**173**(7):473-480. 10.1016/j.neurol.2017.06.009

[38] Fang M, Zhong L, Jin X, Cui R, Yang W, Gao S, et al. Effect of inflammation on the process of stroke rehabilitation and poststroke depression. Frontiers in Psychiatry. 2019;**10**:184

[39] Schaapsmeerders P, Tuladhar AM, Arntz RM, Franssen S, Maaijwee NAM, Rutten-Jacobs LCA, et al. Remote Lower White Matter Integrity Increases the Risk of Long-Term Cognitive Impairment After Ischemic Stroke in Young Adults. Stroke. 2016;**47**(10):251

[40] Mandzia JL, Smith EE, Horton M, Hanly P, Barber, PA, Godzwon C, Coutts SB. Imaging and baseline predictors of cognitive performance in minor ischemic stroke and patients with transient ischemic attack at 90 days. Stroke. 2016;**47**(3);726-731. DOI:10.1161/strokeaha.115.011507

[41] Skrobot OA, Black SE, Chen C, DeCarli C, Erkinjuntti T, Ford GA, et al. Progress toward standardized diagnosis of vascular cognitive impairment: Guidelines from the Vascular Impairment of Cognition Classification Consensus Study. Alzheimer's & Dementia. 2018;**14**(3):280-292. DOI: 10.1016/j.jalz.2017.09.007

[42] Choi BR, Kim DH, Back DB, Kang CH, Moon WJ, Han JS, et al. Characterization of white matter injury in a rat model of chronic cerebral hypoperfusion. Stroke. 2016;**47**(2):542-547. DOI: 10.1161/strokeaha.115.011679

[43] Moulin S, Labreuche J, Bombois S, Rossi C, Boulouis G, Hénon H, et al. Dementia risk after spontaneous intracerebral haemorrhage: A prospective cohort study. Lancet Neurology. 2016;**15**(8):820-829. DOI: 10.1016/s1474-4422(16)00130-7

[44] You S, Wang X, Lindley RI, Robinson T, Anderson CS, Cao Y,

et al. Early cognitive impairment after intracerebral hemorrhage in the INTERACT1 study. Cerebrovascular Diseases. 2017;**44**(5-6):320-324. DOI: 10.1159/000481443

[45] Valenti R, Charidimou A, Xiong L, Boulouis G, Fotiadis P, Ayres A, et al. Visuospatial functioning in cerebral amyloid angiopathy: A Pilot Study. Journal of Alzheimer's Disease. 2017;**56**:1223-1227. DOI: 10.3233/JAD-160927

[46] Banerjee G, Summers M, Chan E, Wilson D, Charidimou A, Cipolotti L, et al. Domain-specific characterisation of early cognitive impairment following spontaneous intracerebral haemorrhage. Journal of the Neurological Sciences. 2018;**391**:25-30. DOI: 10.1016/j.jns.2018.05.015

[47] Wong AMY, Ho CSH, Au TKF, McBride C, Ng AKH, Yip LPW, et al. Reading comprehension, working memory and higher-level language skills in children with SLI and/or dyslexia. Reading and Writing. 2017;**30**:337-361

[48] da Costa L, Shah-Basak PP, Dunkley BT, Robertson AD, Pang EW. Visual working memory encoding and recognition in good outcome aneurysmal subarachnoid patients. Frontiers in Neurology. 2018;**9**:494

[49] Sahyouni R, Goshtasbi K, Mahmoodi A, Tran DK, Chen JW. Chronic subdural hematoma: A perspective on subdural membranes and dementia. World Neurosurgery. 2017;**108**:954-958. DOI: 10.1016/j.wneu.2017.09.063

[50] Cahill-Smith S, Li JM. Oxidative stress, redox signalling and endothelial dysfunction in ageing-related neurodegenerative diseases: A role of NADPH oxidase 2. British Journal of Clinical Pharmacology. 2014;**78**(3):441-453. DOI: 10.1111/bcp.12357

[51] Zlokovic BV. Neurovascular mechanisms of Alzheimer's neurodegeneration. Trends in Neurosciences. 2005;**28**(4):202-208. DOI: 10.1016/j.tins.2005.02.001

[52] Montagne A, Barnes SR, Sweeney MD, Halliday MR, Sagare AP, Zhao Z, et al. Blood-brain barrier breakdown in the aging human hippocampus. Neuron. 2015;**85**(2):296-302. DOI: 10.1016/j.neuron.2014.12.032

[53] Nelson CE, Hakim CH, Ousterout DG, Thakore PI, Moreb EA, Castellanos Rivera RM, et al. In vivo genome editing improves muscle function in a mouse model of Duchenne muscular dystrophy. Science. 2016;**351**(6271):403-407. DOI: 10.1126/science.aad5143

[54] Codex Alimentarius Commission. Standard for Honey. CDX 12-1981. Amended in 2019; pp. 1-8

[55] Crane E, Visscher PK. Honey. In: Resh VH, Cardé RT, editors. Encyclopedia of Insects. 2nd ed. Amsterdam, London: Elsevier; 2009. pp. 459-461. DOI: 10.1016/B978-0-12-374144-8.00130-2

[56] Joshi SR. General overview from honey subsector. In: Renchen K, Sellars-Shrestha S, editors. Honey in Nepal: Approach, Strategy and Intervention for Subsector Promotion. Kathmandu: German Technical Cooperation/Private Sector Promotion-Rural Finance Nepal; 2008. pp. 1-14

[57] Codex Alimentarius Commission. Standard For Honey. 2001; CXS 12-19811 Adopted in 1981. Revised in 1987, 2001

[58] Bogdanov S. Honeys types. In: Harrison C, editor. The Book of Honey. UK: Read Books, Ltd; 2017. pp. 1-6.

[Internet]. Available from: https://www.bee-hexagon.net/english/bee-products/downloads-honey-book/ [Accessed: November 3, 2021]

[59] Rasmussen C, Cameron SA. Global stingless bee phylogeny supports ancient divergence, vicariance, and long distance dispersal. Biological Journal of the Linnean Society. 2010;**99**:206-232

[60] Abd Jalil MA, Kasmuri AR, Haid H. Stingless bee honey, the natural wound healer: A review. Skin Pharmacology and Physiology. 2017;**30**:66-75

[61] Simone-Finstrom M, Spivak M. Propolis and bee health: The natural history and significance of resin use by honey bees. Apidologie. 2010;**41**:295-311

[62] Biluca FC, Braghini F, Gonzaga LV, Costa ACO, Fett R. Physicochemical profiles, minerals, and bioactive compounds of stingless bee honey (Meliponinae). Journal of Food Composition and Analysis. 2016;**50**:61-69

[63] Souza ECA, Menezes C, Flach A. Stingless bee honey (Hymenoptera, Apidae, Meliponini): A review of quality control, chemical profile and biological potential. Apidologie. 2021;**52**:113-132

[64] Kelly N, Farisya MSN, Kumara TK, Marcela P. Species diversity and external nest characteristics of stingless bees in meliponiculture. Pertanika Journal of Tropical Agriculture Science. 2014;**37**(3)

[65] Ramanauskiene K, Stelmakiene A, Briedis V, Ivanauskas L, Jakstas V. The quantitative analysis of biologically active compounds in Lithuanian Honey. Food Chemistry. 2012;**132**:1544-1548

[66] Anklam E. A review of the analytical methods to determine the geographical and botanical origin of honey. Food Chemistry. 1998;**63**(4):549-562

[67] Chuttong B, Chanbang Y, Sringarm K, Burgett M. Physicochemical profiles of stingless bee (Apidae: Meliponini) honey from South East Asia (Thailand). Food Chemistry. 2016;**192**:149-155

[68] Malaysian Standards. Kelulut (Stingless bee) honey-Specification Malaysia Department of Malaysian Standards, 2017; 2683

[69] Alvarez-Suarez JM, Giampieri F, BrenCiani A, Mazzoni L, Gasparrini M, Gonzalez-Paramas AM, et al. *Apis mellifera* vs Meliponanbeecheii cuban polifloral honeys: A comparison base on their physicochemical parameters, chemical composition, and biology properties. LWT: Food Science and Technology. 2018;**87**:272-279

[70] Babarinde GO, Babarinde SA, Adegbola DO, Ajayeoba SI. Effects of /81harvesting methods on physicochemical and microbial qualities of honey. Journal of Food Science and Technology. 2011;**48**(5):628-634

[71] Sancho MT, Mato I, Huidobro JF, Fernandez-Muino MA, Pascual-Mate A. Nonaromatic organic acids of honeys. In: Vit P, Pedro SRM, Roubik DW, editors. Pot-Honey: A Legacy of Stingless Bees. New York: Springer; 2013. pp. 447-458

[72] Almeida-Muradian LB, Stramm KM, Horita A, Barth OM, Freitas AS, Estevinho LM. Comparative study of the physicochemical and palynological characteristics of honey from Melipona subnitida and Apis Mellifera. International Food Science and Technology. 2013;**48**:1698-1706

[73] Solayman M, Islam MA, Paul S, Ali Y, Khalil MI, Alam N, et al. Physicochemical properties, minerals, trace elements, and heavy metals in honey of different origins: A comprehensive review.

Comprehensive Reviews in Food Science and Food Safety. 2016;**15**:219-233

[74] Pasias LN, Kiriakou LK, Proestos C. HMF and diastase acitivity in honeys: A fully and adulteration. Food Chemistry. 2017;**229**:425-431

[75] Nordin A, Sainik NQAV, Chowdhury SR, Saim AB, Idrus RBH. Physicochemical properties of stingless bee honey from around the globe: A comprehensive review. Journal of Food Composition and Analysis. 2018;**73**:91-102

[76] Kek S, Chin N, Yusof Y, Tan S, Chua L. Classification of entomological origin of honey based on its physicochemical and antioxidant properties. International Journal of Food Properties. 2017;**20**(sup3):S2723-S2738

[77] Nishio E, Ribeiro J, Oliveira A, Andrade C, Proni E, Kobayashi R, et al. Antibacterial synergic effect of honey from two stingless bees. Scientific Reports. 2016

[78] Ozbalci B, Boyaci IH, Topcu A, Kadilar C, Tamer U. Rapid analysis of sugars in honey by processing Raman spectrum using chemometric methods and artificial neural networks. Food Chemistry. 2013;**136**(3-4):1444-1452

[79] Budin SB, Jubaidi FF, Azam SNFMN, Yusof NLM, Taib IS, Mohameda J. Kelulut Honey supplementation prevents sperm and testicular oxidative damage in streptozotocin-induced diabetic rats. Jurnal Teknologi. 2017;**79**(3):89-95

[80] National Honey Board (2010). Honey: A reference guide to Nature's sweetener. 2010; p. 1-8 [Internet]. Available from https://honey.com/images/files/Detailed-Nutrition-Information.pdf [Accessed: November 3, 2021]

[81] Boorn KL, Khor YY, Sweetman E, Tan F, Heard TA, Hammer KA. Antimicrobial activity of honey from the stingless bee *Trigona carbonaria* determined by agar diffusion, agar dilution, broth microdilution and time-kill methodology. Journal of Applied Microbiology. 2010;**108**(5):1534-1543

[82] Barakhbah A, Anisah S, Agil S. Honey in the Malay tradition. Malaysian Journal of Medical Sciences. 2007;**14**(1):106

[83] Sabir A, Tabbu CR, Agustiono P, Sosroseno W. Histological analysis of rat dental pulp tissue capped with propolis. Journal of Oral Science. 2005;**47**(3):135-138

[84] Ranneh Y, Akim AM, Hamid HA, Khazaai H, Fadel A, Mahmoud AM. Stingless bee honey protects against lipopolysaccharide induced-chronic subclinical systemic inflammation and oxidative stress by modulating Nrf2, NF-κB and p38 MAPK. Nutrition and Metabolism. 2019;**16**:15-15

[85] Utispan K, Chitkul B, Monthanapisut P, Meesuk L, Pugdee K, Koontongkaew S. Propolis extracted from the stingless bee Trigona sirindhornae inhibited *S. mutans* activity in vitro. Oral Health and Preventive Dentistry. 2017b;**15**(3):279-284

[86] Kafaween M, Abu Bakar MH, Khan R. In vitro investigation on the effectiveness of Trigona honey against biofilm formation by *Escherichia coli*. EC Microbiology. 2020;**16**:83-89

[87] Saiful Yazan L, Muhamad Zali MFS, Mohd Ali R, Zainal NA, Esa N, Sapuan S, et al. Chemopreventive properties and toxicity of Kelulut honey in *Sprague Dawley* rats induced with Azoxymethane. BioMed Research International. 2016;**2016**:4036926

[88] Ahmad F, Seerangan P, Mustafa MZ, Osman ZF, Abdullah JM, Idris Z. Anti-cancer properties of *Heterotrigona itama* sp. Honey Via induction of apoptosis in malignant glioma cells. Malays Journal of Medical Sciences. 2019;**26**(2):30-39

[89] Selvaraju K, Vikram P, Soon JM, Krishnan KT, Mohammed A. Melissopalynological, physicochemical and antioxidant properties of honey from West Coast of Malaysia. Journal of Food Science and Technology. 2019;**56**(5):2508-2521

[90] Al-Hatamleh MA, Boer JC, Wilson KL, Plebanski M, Mohamud R, Mustafa MZ. Antioxidant based medicinal properties of stingless bee products: Recent progress and future direction. Biomolecules. 2020

[91] Mohd Sairazi NS, Sirajudeen KNS, Muzaimi M, Mummedy S, Asari MA, Sulaiman SA. Tualang honey reduced neuroinflammation and caspase-3 activity in rat brain after kainic acid-induced status epilepticus. Evidence-based Complementary and Alternative Medicine. 2018;**2018**:7287820

[92] Mustafa MZ, Yaacob NS, Sulaiman SA. Reinventing the honey industry: Opportunities of the stingless bee. The Malaysian Journal of Medical Sciences. 2018;**25**(4):1-5. DOI: 10.21315/mjms2018.25.4.1

[93] Oyefuga O, Ajani E, Salau B, Agboola F, Adebawo O. Honey consumption and its anti-ageing potency in white Wister albino rats. Scholarly Journal of Biological Science. 2012;**1**(2):15-19

[94] Zulkhairi Amin FA, Sabri S, Mohammad SM, Ismail M, Chan KW, Ismail N, et al. Therapeutic properties of stingless bee honey in comparison with European bee honey. Advances in Pharmacological Sciences. 2018:6179596. DOI: 10.1155/2018/6179596

[95] Mijanur Rahman M, Gan SH, Khalil MI. Neurological effects of honey: Current and future prospects. Evidence-based Complementary and Alternative Medicine. 2014:958721

[96] He X-L, Wang Y-H, Bi M-G, Du G-H. Chrysin improves cognitive deficits and brain damage induced by chronic cerebral hypoperfusion in rats. European Journal of Pharmacology. 2012;**680**(1):41-48

[97] Pietá Dias C, Martins de Lima MN, Presti-Torres J, Dornelles A, Garcia VA, Siciliani Scalco F, et al. Memantine reduces oxidative damage and enhances long-term recognition memory in aged rats. Neuroscience. 2007;**146**(4):1719-1725

[98] Isuzugawa K, Ogihara Y, Inoue M. Different generation of inhibitors against gallic acid-induced apoptosis produces different sensitivity to gallic acid. Biological and Pharmaceutical Bulletin. 2001;**24**(3):249-253

[99] Mansouri MT, Farbood Y, Sameri MJ, Sarkaki A, Naghizadeh B, Rafeirad M. Neuroprotective effects of oral gallic acid against oxidative stress induced by 6-hydroxydopamine in rats. Food Chemistry. 2013;**138**(2-3):1028-1033

[100] Zulkhairi Amin FA, Sabri S, Mohammad SM, Ismail M, Chan KW, Ismail N, et al. Therapeutic properties of stingless bee honey in comparison with European bee honey. Advances in Pharmacological Sciences. 2018:6179596. DOI: 10.1155/2018/6179596

[101] Korani MS, Farbood Y, Sarkaki A, Fathi Moghaddam H, Taghi Mansouri M. Protective effects of gallic acid against chronic cerebral hypoperfusion-induced

cognitive deficit and brain oxidative damage in rats. European Journal of Pharmacology. 2014;**733**:62-67

[102] Gao J, Hu J, Hu D, Yang X. A role of gallic acid in oxidative damage diseases: A comprehensive review. Natural Product Communications. 2019;**14**(8):1-9

[103] Ferguson LR, Zhu S-T, Harris PJ. Antioxidant and antigenotoxic effects of plant cell wall hydroxycinnamic acids in cultured HT-29 cells. Molecular Nutrition & Food Research. 2005;**49**(6): 585-593

[104] Vauzour D, Corona G, Spencer JPE. Caffeic acid, tyrosol and p-coumaric acid are potent inhibitors of 5-S-cysteinyl-dopamine induced neurotoxicity. Archives of Biochemistry and Biophysics. 2010;**501**(1):106-111. DOI: https://doi.org/10.1016/j.abb.2010.03.016

[105] Takao K, Toda K, Saito T, Sugita Y. Synthesis of amide and ester derivatives of cinnamic acid and its analogs: Evaluation of their free radical scavenging and monoamine oxidase and cholinesterase inhibitory activities. Chemical & Pharmaceutical Bulletin (Tokyo). 2017;**65**(11):1020-1027

[106] Ghosh A, Sarkar S, Mandal AK, Das N. Neuroprotective role of nanoencapsulated quercetin in combating ischemia-reperfusion induced neuronal damage in young and aged rats. PLoS One. 2013;**8**(4):e57735

[107] Xia SF, Xie ZX, Qiao Y, Li LR, Cheng XR, Tang X, et al. Differential effects of quercetin on hippocampus-dependent learning and memory in mice fed with different diets related with oxidative stress. Physiology & Behavior. 2015;**138**:325-331

[108] Bhullar KS, Rupasinghe HPV. Polyphenols: Multipotent therapeutic agents in neurodegenerative diseases. Oxidative Medicine and Cellular Longevity. 2013:891748

[109] Costa LG, Garrick JM, Roquè PJ, Pellacani C. Mechanisms of neuroprotection by quercetin: Counteracting oxidative stress and more. Oxidative Medicine and Cellular Longevity. 2016:2986796

[110] Paula P-C, Angelica Maria S-G, Luis C-H, Gloria Patricia C-G. Preventive effect of quercetin in a triple transgenic Alzheimer's disease mice model. Molecules. 2019;**24**(12):2287

[111] Zhang X-W, Chen J-Y, Ouyang D, Lu J-H. Quercetin in animal models of Alzheimer's disease: A systematic review of preclinical studies. International Journal of Molecular Sciences. 2020;**21**(2):493

[112] Bernatoniene J, Kopustinskiene DM. The role of catechins in cellular responses to oxidative stress. Molecules. 2018;**23**(4):965

[113] Sutherland BA, Rahman RMA, Appleton I. Mechanisms of action of green tea catechins, with a focus on ischemia-induced neurodegeneration. The Journal of Nutritional Biochemistry. 2006;**17**(5):291-306

[114] Lee S-R, Suh S-I, Kim S-P. Protective effects of the green tea polyphenol (−)-epigallocatechin gallate against hippocampal neuronal damage after transient global ischemia in gerbils. Neuroscience Letters. 2000;**287**(3):191-194

[115] Lee H, Bae JH, Lee S-R. Protective effect of green tea polyphenol EGCG against neuronal damage and brain edema after unilateral cerebral ischemia in gerbils. Journal of Neuroscience Research. 2004;**77**(6):892-900

[116] Unno K, Takabayashi F, Oku N. Improvement in brain function and oxidative damage of aged senescence-accelerated mice by green tea catechins. International Congress Series. 2004;**1260**:409-412

[117] Liu S-Q, Su F, Fang L-M, Xia Q, Zhang X. Protective effect of apigenin on neurons against oxygen-glucose deprivation/reperfusion induced injury. The FASEB Journal. 2010;**24**(S1):604.615-604.615. DOI: https://doi.org/10.1096/fasebj.24.1_supplement.604.15

[118] Han J-Y, Ahn S-Y, Kim C-S, Yoo S-K, Kim S-K, Kim H-C, et al. Protection of apigenin against kainate-induced excitotoxicity by anti-oxidative effects. Biological and Pharmaceutical Bulletin. 2012;**35**(9):1440-1446

[119] Pang Q, Zhao Y, Chen X, Zhao K, Zhai Q, Tu F. Apigenin protects the brain against ischemia/reperfusion injury via Caveolin-1/VEGF in vitro and in vivo. Oxidative Medicine and Cellular Longevity. 2018:7017204

[120] Ling C, Lei C, Zou M, Cai X, Xiang Y, Xie Y, et al. Neuroprotective effect of apigenin against cerebral ischemia/reperfusion injury. Journal of International Medical Research. 2020;**48**(9)

[121] Tolba MF, Omar HA, Azab SS, Khalifa AE, Abdel-Naim AB, Abdel-Rahman SZ. Caffeic acid phenethyl ester: A review of its antioxidant activity, protective effects against ischemia-reperfusion injury and drug adverse reactions. Critical Reviews in Food Science and Nutrition. 2016;**56**(13):2183-2190

[122] Hwang SA, Kim CD, Lee WS. Caffeic acid phenethyl ester protects against photothrombotic cortical ischemic injury in mice. Korean Journal of Physiology and Pharmacology. 2018;**22**(1):101-110

[123] Filomeni G, Graziani I, De Zio D, Dini L, Centonze D, Rotilio G, et al. Neuroprotection of kaempferol by autophagy in models of rotenone-mediated acute toxicity: Possible implications for Parkinson's disease. Neurobiology of Aging. 2012;**33**(4):767-785

[124] Yu L, Chen C, Wang L-F, Kuang X, Liu K, Zhang H, et al. Neuroprotective effect of kaempferol glycosides against brain injury and neuroinflammation by inhibiting the activation of NF-κB and STAT3 in transient focal stroke. PloS One. 2013;**8**(2):e55839-e55839

[125] Li W-H, Cheng X, Yang Y-L, Liu M, Zhang S-S, Wang Y-H, et al. Kaempferol attenuates neuroinflammation and blood brain barrier dysfunction to improve neurological deficits in cerebral ischemia/reperfusion rats. Brain Research. 2019;**1722**:146361

[126] Park S-H, Sim Y-B, Han P-L, Lee J-K, Suh H-W. Antidepressant-like effect of Kaempferol and Quercitirin, isolated from Opuntia ficus-indica var. saboten. Experimental Neurobiology. 2010;**19**(1):30

[127] Cipollini V et al. Emerging biomarkers in vascular cognitive impairment and dementia: From pathophysiological pathways to clinical application. International Journal of Molecular Sciences. 2019;**20**(11):2812

[128] Schuitemaker A et al. Inflammatory markers in AD and MCI patients with different biomarker profiles. Neurobiology of Aging. 2010;**30**(11):1885-1889

[129] Meo SA et al. Role of honey in modern medicine. Saudi Journal of Biological Sciences. 2017;**24**(5):975-978

[130] Azman KF, Zakaria R. Honey as an antioxidant therapy to reduce cognitive aging. Iranian Journal of Basic Medical Sciences. 2019

[131] Engwa GA. Free radicals and the role of phytochemicals as antioxidants against. Oxidative Stress-Related Diseases. 2018;**49**

[132] Su F, Xu W. Enhancing brain plasticity to promote stroke recovery. Frontiers in Neurology. 2020;**11**:1422

[133] Cai M, Shin BY, Kim DH, et al. Neuroprotective effects of additional herbal prescription on transient cerebral global ischemia in gerbils. Journtraal of Ethnopharmacology. 2011;**138**(3):723-730

[134] Mustafa MZ, Zulkifli FN, Fernandez I, Mariatulqabtiah AR, Sangu M, Nor Azfa J, et al. Stingless bee honey improves spatial memory in mice, probably associated with brain-derived neurotrophic factor (BDNF) and inositol 1,4,5-triphosphate receptor Type 1 (*Itpr1*) genes. Evidence-based Complementary and Alternative Medicine. 2019;**2019**:8258307. DOI: 10.1155/2019/8258307

[135] Al-Hatamleh MAI, Hussin TMAR, Taib WRW, Ismail I. The brain-derived neurotrophic factor (BDNF) gene Val66Met (rs6265) polymorphism and stress among preclinical medical students in Malaysia. Journal of Taibah University Medical Sciences. 2019;**14**(5):431-438. DOI: 10.1016/j.jtumed.2019.09.003

[136] Sun M-S, Jin H, Sun X, Huang S, Zhang F-L, Guo Z-N, et al. Free radical damage in ischemia-reperfusion injury: An obstacle in acute ischemic stroke after revascularization therapy. Oxidative Medicine and Cellular Longevity. 2018;**2018**:3804979

[137] Schliebs R, Arendt T. The cholinergic system in aging and neuronal degeneration. Behavioural Brain Research. 2011;**221**(2):555-563. DOI: 10.1016/j.bbr.2010.11.058

[138] Koc AN, Silici S, Kasap F, Hormet-Oz HT, Mavus-Buldu H, Ercal BD. Antifungal activity of the honeybee products against Candida spp and Trichosporon spp. Journal of Medicinal Food. 2011;**14**:128-134

[139] Carlson AB, Kraus GP. Physiology, Cholinergic Receptors *StatPearls*. Treasure Island (FL): StatPearls Publishing LLC; 2021

[140] Jabir NR, Khan FR, Tabrez S. Cholinesterase targeting by polyphenols: A therapeutic approach for the treatment of Alzheimer's disease. CNS Neuroscience & Therapeutics. 2018;**24**(9):753-762. DOI: 10.1111/cns.12971

[141] Camps P, El Achab R, Morral J, Muñoz-Torrero D, Badia A, Baños JE, Luque FJ. New tacrine-huperzine A hybrids (huprines): Highly potent tight-binding acetylcholinesterase inhibitors of interest for the treatment of Alzheimer's disease. Journal of Medicinal Chemistry, 2000;**43**(24):4657-4666. DOI: 10.1021/jm000980y

[142] Sharma K. Cholinesterase inhibitors as Alzheimer's therapeutics (Review). Molecular Medicine Reports. 2019;**20**(2):1479-1487. DOI: 10.3892/mmr.2019.10374

[143] Xing S-H, Zhu C-X, Zhang R, An L. Huperzine A in the treatment of Alzheimer's disease and vascular dementia: A meta-analysis. Evidence-based Complementary and Alternative Medicine. 2014;**2014**:363985. DOI: 10.1155/2014/363985